2013

Guide to Occupational Exposure Values

Compiled by
ACGIH®

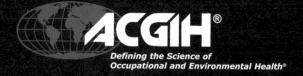

ACGIH®
Defining the Science of
Occupational and Environmental Health®

Signature Publications

ISBN: 978-1-607260-60-8

Published in the United States of America by
ACGIH®
1330 Kemper Meadow Drive
Cincinnati, Ohio 45240-4148
www.acgih.org

Printed in the United States

2013

Guide to Occupational Exposure Values

Compiled by
ACGIH®

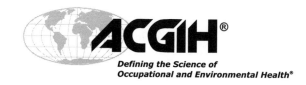

ACGIH®
Defining the Science of
Occupational and Environmental Health®

Signature Publications

The *Guide to Occupational Exposure Values* is a readily accessible reference for comparison of published values from ACGIH®; the U.S. Occupational Safety and Health Administration (OSHA); the U.S. National Institute for Occupational Safety and Health (NIOSH); Deutsche Forschungsgemeinschaft (DFG), Federal Republic of Germany, Commission for the Investigation of Health Hazards of Chemical Compounds in the Work Area; and the American Industrial Hygiene Association (AIHA). Provided below are the sources of the values cited in this *Guide*, including publication dates, and the uniform resource locator (URL) if verified online. November 2012 was the date of online verification.

- ACGIH® Threshold Limit Values (TLVs®) for Chemical Substances

  ○ *2013 TLVs® and BEIs®: Threshold Limit Values for Chemical Substances and Physical Agents and Biological Exposure Indices.* ACGIH®, Cincinnati, OH (2013).

- OSHA Permissible Exposure Limits (PELs)

  ○ Title 29, Code of Federal Regulations, Part 1910.1000-1910.1200, Air Contaminants, Final Rule, specified in Tables Z-1, Z-2, and Z-3; Federal Register 58:35338-35351, June 30, 1993; corrected in Federal Register 58:40191, July 27, 1993; amended in Federal Register 60:9624, February 21, 1995; Federal Register 60:33343, June 28, 1995; corrected in Federal Register 60:33984, June 29, 1995; Federal Register 62:42018, August 4, 1997; and subsequent corrections/amendments/proposals through Federal Register 71:10373, February 28, 2006. Reviewed at http://www.osha.gov/pls/oshaweb/owadisp.show_document?p_table=STANDARDS&p_id=9992.

- NIOSH Recommended Exposure Limits (RELs)

  ○ NIOSH Pocket Guide to Chemical Hazards: Introduction. Available online at: http://www.cdc.gov/niosh/npg/pgintrod.html (Updated 2010).

  ○ *See also*: Ludwig HR; Cairelli SG; Whalen JJ (Eds): Documentation for Immediately Dangerous to Life or Health Concentrations (IDLH): Introduction. NTIS Pub. No. PB-94-195047 (1994). Available online at: http://www.cdc.gov/niosh/idlh/idlhintr.html.

- DFG Maximum Concentrations at the Workplace (MAKs)

  ○ List of MAK and BAT Values 2012: Maximum Concentrations and Biological Tolerance Values at the Workplace. Report No. 47. Commission for the Investigation of Health Hazards of Chemical Compounds in the Work Area. Wiley-VCH Verlag GmbH & Co. KGaA, Weinheim, FRG (July 1, 2012).

- AIHA Workplace Environmental Exposure Levels (WEELs™)

  ○ 2011 current WEEL® values. AIHA Guideline Foundation, Fairfax, VA. Available online at http://www.aiha.org/insideaiha/GuidelineDevelopment/Weel/Documents/2011%20WEEL%20Values.pdf.

The *Guide* also includes those carcinogens found in the occupational environment that are identified by the above organizations and by the U.S. Environmental Protection Agency (EPA), the International Agency for Research on Cancer (IARC), and the U.S. National Toxicology Program (NTP). In addition to those sources cited above, the following were also used in preparing this *Guide* and were reviewed in November 2012.

- U.S. EPA Integrated Risk Information System (IRIS) database. A–Z List of Substances. Online at: http://cfpub.epa.gov/ncea/iris/index.cfm?fuseaction=iris.showsubstancelist.

- Agents Classified by the IARC Monographs, Volumes 1–102. IARC, Lyon, France (1987–2012). Available online at: http://monographs.iarc.fr/ENG/Classification/index.php (Updated November 7, 2012).

- Report on Carcinogens, 12th Ed., U.S. Department of Health and Human Services, Public Health Service, National Toxicology Program, Research Triangle Park, NC. Available online at: http://ntp.niehs.nih.gov/ntp/roc/twelfth/roc12.pdf (Updated 2011).

The *Guide to Occupational Exposure Values* is intended as a companion document to the ACGIH® annual *Threshold Limit Values for Chemical Substances and Physical Agents and Biological Exposure Indices* (*TLVs® and BEIs®*) book, specifically the section on TLVs® for Chemical Substances in the Work Environment.

The following pages provide "Definitions, Abbreviations, Terms, and Coding," the MAK "Peak Exposure Limitation Categories," the MAK "Pregnancy Risk Group Classifications," and the MAK "Germ Cell Mutagens Classifications."

Editor's note: The double entries that were previously included in this publication were eliminated effective with the 2006 edition. The entry in this publication will correspond to that carried in the *TLVs® and BEIs®* book, e.g., 2-butoxyethanol rather than ethylene glycol monobutyl ether. When ACGIH® does not recommend a TLV® and two or more jurisdictions (e.g., MAK and IARC) list a chemical substance with separate synonyms, ACGIH® will generally use the ChemIDplus database available on the ToxNet website (http://toxnet.nlm.nih.gov/) maintained by the U.S. National Library of Medicine. ChemIDplus is a database of over 370,000 chemicals, which contains names and synonyms as well as chemical formulae and structures. Whichever synonym ChemIDplus uses as the primary name attached to a specific CAS number is the name generally listed in this publication. In all cases, the removed synonym is listed with its primary entry and with its respective CAS number in the CAS Number Index section of this publication.

Carcinogenicity Categories

U.S. Environmental Protection Agency (EPA)

NOTE: The rationale and methods used to develop the carcinogenicity classifications EPA-A through EPA-E are found in the 1986 *Risk Assessment Guidelines* (EPA/600/8-87/045). The categories, EPA-K, EPA-L, EPA-CBD, and EPA-UL, were developed under the 1996 *Proposed Guidelines for Carcinogen Risk Assessment* (*Federal Register* 61[79]:17960-18011, April 23, 1996). Further to its updating of risk assessment guidelines, EPA issued a revised draft *Guidelines for Carcinogen Risk Assessment* (NCEA-F-0644; July 1999), which resulted in slightly different descriptors. In 2005, the agency published the final version of *Guidelines for Carcinogen Risk Assessment* (EPA/630/P-03-001 B), which contained refined descriptors for summarizing weight of evidence for human carcinogenic potential. All four risk assessment guidelines may be found online at: **http://www.epa.gov/riskassessment/guidance.htm**. In all instances, the user is referred to the online IRIS Guidance Documents found on the EPA website: **http://www.epa.gov/ncea/iris/backgrd.html** and the online Toxicological Reviews and Support Documents available at: **http://cfpub.epa.gov/ncea/iris/index.cfm?fuseaction=iris.showToxDocs** for further carcinogenicity discussion and for information on long-term toxic effects other than carcinogenicity. In all cases, the most current carcinogenicity assessment will be listed in this publication.

EPA-A: Human Carcinogen — Sufficient evidence from epidemiologic studies to support a causal association between exposure and cancer.

-B: Probable Human Carcinogen — Weight of evidence of human carcinogenicity based on epidemiologic studies is limited; agents for which weight of evidence of carcinogenicity based on animal studies is sufficient.

Two subgroups:

-B1: Limited evidence of carcinogenicity from epidemiologic studies.

-B2: Sufficient evidence from animal studies; inadequate evidence or no data from epidemiologic studies.

-C: Possible Human Carcinogen — Limited evidence of carcinogenicity in animals in the absence of human data.

-D: Not Classifiable as to Human Carcinogenicity — Inadequate human and animal evidence of carcinogenicity or no data are available.

-E: Evidence of Noncarcinogenicity for Humans — No evidence for carcinogenicity in at least two adequate animal tests in different species or in both adequate epidemiologic and animal studies.

Under the 1996 Draft Guidelines, when the available tumor effects and other key data are adequate to demonstrate carcinogenic potential convincingly for humans, EPA-K or EPA-L are appropriate descriptors.

EPA-K: Known Human Carcinogens — Agents *known* to be carcinogenic in humans based on either epidemiologic evidence or a combination of epidemiologic and experimental evidence, demonstrating causality between human exposure and cancer;

OR

Agents that should be treated *as if* they were *known* human carcinogens, based on a combination of epidemiologic data showing a plausible causal association (not demonstrating it definitively) and strong experimental evidence.

-L: Likely to Produce Cancer in Humans — Agents that are *likely* to produce cancer in humans due to the production or anticipated production of tumors by modes of action that are relevant or assumed to be relevant to human carcinogenicity. Modifying descriptors for particularly high or low ranking in the "known/likely" group can be applied based on scientific judgment and experience and are as follows:

- Agents that are *likely* to produce cancer in humans based on data that are at the high end of the weights of evidence typical of this group.

- Agents that are *likely* to produce cancer in humans based on data that are at the low end of the weights of evidence typical of this group.

-CBD: Cannot Be Determined — This descriptor is appropriate when available tumor effects or other key data are suggestive or conflicting or limited in quantity and, thus, are not adequate to convincingly demonstrate carcinogenic potential for humans. In general, further agent specific and generic research and testing are needed to be able to describe human carcinogenic potential. The descriptor *cannot be determined* is used with a subdescriptor that captures the rationale:

- Agents whose carcinogenic potential *cannot be determined*, but for which there is suggestive evidence that raises concern for carcinogenic effects.

- Agents whose carcinogenic potential cannot be determined because the existing evidence is composed of *conflicting data* (e.g., some evidence is suggestive of carcinogenic effects, but other equally pertinent evidence does not confirm any concern).

- Agents whose carcinogenic potential *cannot be determined* because there are inadequate data to perform an assessment.

- Agents whose carcinogenic potential *cannot be determined* because no data are available to perform an assessment.

-NL: Not Likely to be Carcinogenic in Humans — This descriptor is appropriate when experimental evidence is satisfactory for deciding that there is no basis for human hazard concern, as follows (in the absence of human data suggesting a potential for cancer effects):

- Agents *not likely* to be carcinogenic to humans because they have been evaluated in at least two well-conducted studies in two appropriate animal species without demonstrating carcinogenic effects.

- Agents *not likely* to be carcinogenic to humans because they have been appropriately evaluated in animals and show only carcinogenic effects that have been shown not to be relevant to humans (e.g., showing only effects in the male rat kidney due to accumulation of α_2u-globulin).

- Agents *not likely* to be carcinogenic to humans when carcinogenicity is dose or route dependent. For instance, not likely below a certain dose range (categorized as *likely* above that range) or *not likely* by a certain route of exposure (may be categorized as likely by another route of exposure). To qualify, agents will have been appropriately evaluated in animal studies and the only effects show a dose range or route limitation or a route limitation is otherwise shown by empirical data.

Under the 1999 revised draft Guidelines, the following descriptors were issued; however, the descriptors are only presented in the context of a weight-of-evidence-narrative. [*Editor's note*: The "short hand" used within this *Guide* (e.g., EPA-K) to indicate descriptors used within the 1996 and 1999 draft Guidelines were developed to accommodate the page format only.] The reader is referred to the current EPA evaluation for a complete discussion of substance in question.

EPA-CaH: Carcinogenic to Humans — This descriptor is appropriate when there is convincing epidemiologic evidence demonstrating causality between human exposure and cancer. This descriptor is also appropriate when there is an absence of conclusive epidemiologic evidence to clearly establish a cause and effect relationship between human exposure and cancer, but there is compelling evidence of carcinogenicity in animals and mechanistic information in animals and humans demonstrating similar mode(s) of carcinogenic action. It is used when all of the following conditions are met:

- There is evidence in a human population(s) of association of exposure to the agent with cancer, but not enough to show a causal association;

- There is extensive evidence of carcinogenicity;

- The mode(s) of carcinogenic action and associated key events have been identified in animals; and

- The key events that precede the cancer response in animals have been observed in the human population(s) that also show evidence of an association of exposure to the agent with cancer.

-L: Likely to be Carcinogenic to Humans — This descriptor is appropriate when the available tumor effects and other key data are adequate to demonstrate carcinogenic potential to humans. Adequate data are within a spectrum. At one end is evidence for an association between human exposure to the agent and cancer and strong experimental evidence of carcinogenicity in animals; at the other, with no human data, the weight of experimental evidence shows animal carcinogenicity by a mode or modes of action that are relevant or assumed to be relevant to humans.

-S: Suggestive Evidence of Carcinogenicity, but Not Sufficient to Assess Human Carcinogenic Potential — This descriptor is appropriate when the evidence from human or animal data is suggestive of carcinogenicity, which raises a concern for carcinogenic effects but is judged not sufficient for a conclusion as to human carcinogenic potential. Examples of such evidence may include: a marginal increase in tumors that may be exposure-related, or evidence is observed only in a single study, or the only evidence is limited to certain high background tumors in one sex of one species. Dose–response assessment is not indicated for these agents. Further studies would be needed to determine human carcinogenic potential.

-I: Data are Inadequate for an Assessment of Human Carcinogenic Potential — This descriptor is used when available data are judged inadequate to perform an assessment. This includes a case when there is a lack of pertinent or useful data or when existing evidence is conflicting, e.g., some evidence is suggestive of carcinogenic effects, but other equally pertinent evidence does not confirm a concern.

-NL: Not Likely to be Carcinogenic to Humans — This descriptor is used when the available data are considered robust for deciding that there is no basis for human hazard concern. The judgment may be based on the following:

- Extensive human experience that demonstrates lack of carcinogenic effect (e.g., phenobarbital).

- Animal evidence that demonstrates lack of carcinogenic effect in at least two well-designed and well-conducted studies in two appropriate animal species (in the absence of human data suggesting a potential for cancer effects).

- Extensive experimental evidence showing that the only carcinogenic effects observed in animals are not considered relevant to humans (e.g., showing only effects in the male rat kidney due to accumulation of α_2u-globulin).

- Evidence that carcinogenic effects are not likely by a particular route of exposure (Section 2.3.3.).

- Evidence that carcinogenic effects are not anticipated below a defined dose range.

Under the 2005 *Guidelines for Carcinogen Risk Assessment* (EPA/630/P-03/001 B), the following descriptors were issued; however, the descriptors are only presented in the context of a weight-of-evidence-narrative. [*Editor's note*: The "short hand" (e.g., EPA-CaH) used within this *Guide* to indicate the 2005 descriptors was developed to accommodate the page format of this *Guide* only.] The reader is referred to the individual IRIS evaluation for a complete discussion of the substance in question.

EPA-CaH: Carcinogenic to Humans — This descriptor indicates strong evidence of human carcinogenicity. It covers different combinations of evidence.

- This descriptor is appropriate when there is convincing epidemiologic evidence of a causal association between human exposure and cancer.

- Exceptionally, this descriptor may be equally appropriate with a lesser weight of epidemiologic evidence that is strengthened by other lines of evidence. It can be used when all of the following conditions are met: (a) there is strong evidence of an association between human exposure and either cancer or the key precursor events of the agent's mode of action but not enough for a causal association, and (b) there is extensive evidence of carcinogenicity in animals, and (c) the mode(s) of carcinogenic action and associated key precursor events have been identified in animals, and (d) there is strong evidence that the key precursor events that precede the cancer response in animals are anticipated to occur in humans and progress to tumors, based on available biological information. In this case, the narrative includes a summary of both the experimental and epidemio-logic information on mode of action and also an indication of the relative weight that each source of information carries, e.g., based on human information, based on limited human and extensive animal experiments.

-L: Likely to Be Carcinogenic to Humans — This descriptor is appropriate when the weight of the evidence is adequate to demonstrate carcinogenic potential to humans but does not reach the weight of evidence for the "Carcinogenic to Humans" descriptor. Adequate evidence consistent with this descriptor covers a broad spectrum. As stated previously, the use of the term "likely " as a weight of evidence descriptor does not correspond to a quantifiable probability. The examples below are meant to represent the broad range of data combinations that are covered by this descriptor; they are illustrative and provide neither a checklist nor a limitation for the data that might support use of this descriptor. Moreover, additional information, e.g., on mode of action, might change the choice of descriptor for the illustrated examples. Supporting data for this descriptor may include:

- an agent demonstrating a plausible (but not definitively causal) association between human exposure and cancer, in most cases with some supporting biological, experimental evidence, though not necessarily carcinogenicity data from animal experiments;

- an agent that has tested positive in animal experiments in more than one species, sex, strain, site, or exposure route, with or without evidence of carcinogenicity in humans;

- a positive tumor study that raises additional biological concerns beyond that of a statistically significant result, for example, a high degree of malignancy, or an early age at onset;

- a rare animal tumor response in a single experiment that is assumed to be relevant to humans; or

- a positive tumor study that is strengthened by other lines of evidence, for example, either plausible (but not definitively causal) association between human exposure and cancer <u>or</u> evidence that the agent or an important metabolite causes events generally known to be associated with tumor formation (such as DNA reactivity or effects on cell growth control) likely to be related to the tumor response in this case.

-S: Suggestive Evidence of Carcinogenic Potential — This descriptor of the database is appropriate when the weight of evidence is suggestive of carcinogenicity; a concern for potential carcinogenic effects in humans is raised, but the data are judged not sufficient for a stronger conclusion. This descriptor covers a spectrum of evidence associated with varying levels of concern for carcinogenicity, ranging from a positive cancer result in the only study on an agent to a single positive cancer result in an extensive database that includes negative studies in other species. Depending on the extent of the database, additional studies may or may not provide further insights. Some examples include:

- a small, and possibly not statistically significant, increase in tumor incidence observed in a single animal or human study that does not reach the weight of evidence for the descriptor "Likely to Be Carcinogenic to Humans." The study generally would not be contradicted by other studies of equal quality in the same population group or experimental system (*see* discussions of *conflicting evidence* and differing results, below);

- a small increase in a tumor with a high background rate in that sex and strain, when there is some but insufficient evidence that the observed tumors may be due to intrinsic factors that cause background tumors and not due to the agent being assessed. (When there is a high background rate of a specific tumor in animals of a particular sex and strain, then there

may be biological factors operating independently of the agent being assessed that could be responsible for the development of the observed tumors.) In this case, the reasons for determining that the tumors are not due to the agent are explained;

- evidence of a positive response in a study whose power, design, or conduct limits the ability to draw a confident conclusion (but does not make the study fatally flawed), but where the carcinogenic potential is strengthened by other lines of evidence (such as structure-activity relationships); or

- a statistically significant increase at one dose only, but no significant response at the other doses and no overall trend.

-II: Inadequate Information to Assess Carcinogenic Potential — This descriptor of the database is appropriate when available data are judged inadequate for applying one of the other descriptors. Additional studies generally would be expected to provide further insights. Some examples include:

- little or no pertinent information;

- conflicting evidence, that is, some studies provide evidence of carcinogenicity but other studies of equal quality in the same sex and strain are negative. *Differing results*, that is, positive results in some studies and negative results in one or more different experimental systems, do not constitute *conflicting evidence*, as the term is used here. Depending on the overall weight of evidence, differing results can be considered either suggestive evidence or likely evidence; or

- negative results that are not sufficiently robust for the descriptor, "Not Likely to Be Carcinogenic to Humans."

-NL: Not Likely to Be Carcinogenic to Humans — This descriptor is appropriate when the available data are considered robust for deciding that there is no basis for human hazard concern. In some instances, there can be positive results in experimental animals when there is strong, consistent evidence that each mode of action in experimental animals does not operate in humans. In other cases, there can be convincing evidence in both humans and animals that the agent is not carcinogenic. The judgment may be based on data such as:

- animal evidence that demonstrates lack of carcinogenic effect in both sexes in well-designed and well-conducted studies in at least two appropriate animal species (in the absence of other animal or human data suggesting a potential for cancer effects);

- convincing and extensive experimental evidence showing that the only carcinogenic effects observed in animals are not relevant to humans;

- convincing evidence that carcinogenic effects are not likely by a particular exposure route; or

- convincing evidence that carcinogenic effects are not likely below a defined dose range.

The "Not Likely" descriptor applies only to the circumstances supported by the data. For example, an agent may be "Not Likely to Be Carcinogenic" by one route but not necessarily by another. In those cases that have positive animal experiment(s) but the results are judged to be not relevant to humans, the narrative discusses why the results are not relevant.

International Agency for Research on Cancer (IARC)

IARC-1: Carcinogenic to Humans — The exposure circumstance entails exposures that are carcinogenic to humans. This category is used when there is *sufficient evidence* of carcinogenicity in humans. Exceptionally, an agent (mixture) may be placed in the category when evidence in humans is less than sufficient but there is *sufficient evidence* of carcinogenicity in experimental animals and strong evidence in exposed humans that the agent (mixture) acts through a relevant mechanism of carcinogenicity.

-2A: Probably Carcinogenic to Humans — The exposure circumstance entails exposures that are probably carcinogenic to humans. This category is used when there is *limited evidence* of carcinogenicity in humans and sufficient evidence of carcinogenicity in experimental animals. In some cases, an agent (mixture) may be classified in this category when there is inadequate evidence of carcinogenicity in humans and *sufficient evidence* of carcinogenicity in experimental animals and strong evidence that the carcinogenesis is mediated by a mechanism that also operates in humans. Exceptionally, an agent, mixture, or exposure circumstance may be classified in this category solely on the basis of limited evidence of carcinogenicity in humans.

-2B: Possibly Carcinogenic to Humans — The exposure circumstance entails exposures that are possibly carcinogenic to humans. This category is used for agents, mixtures, and exposure circumstances for which there is *limited evidence* of carcinogenicity in humans and less than *sufficient evidence* of carcinogenicity in experimental animals. It may also be used when there is *inadequate evidence* of carcinogenicity in humans but there is *sufficient evidence* of carcinogenicity in experimental animals. In some instances, an agent, mixture, or exposure circumstance for which there is inadequate evidence of carcinogenicity in humans but *limited evidence* of carcinogenicity in experimental animals together with supporting evidence from other relevant data may be placed in the group.

-3: Unclassifiable as to Carcinogenicity in Humans — This category is used most commonly for agents, mixtures, and exposure circumstances for which the evidence of carcinogenicity is inadequate in humans and inadequate or limited in experimental animals. Exceptionally, agents (mixtures) for which the evidence of carcinogenicity is inadequate in humans but sufficient in experimental animals may be placed in this category when there is strong evidence that the mechanism of carcinogenicity in experimental animals does not operate in humans. Agents, mixtures, and exposure circumstances that do not fall into any other group are also placed in this category.

-4: Probably Not Carcinogenic to Humans — This category is used for agents or mixtures for which there is *evidence suggesting lack of carcinogenicity* in humans and in experimental animals. In some instances, agents or mixtures for which there is *inadequate evidence* of carcinogenicity in humans but *evidence suggesting lack of carcinogenicity* in experimental animals, consistently and strongly supported by a broad range of other relevant data, may be classified in this group.

German MAK Commission

MAK-1: Substances that cause cancer in man and can be assumed to make a significant contribution to cancer risk. Epidemiological studies provide adequate evidence of a positive correlation between the exposure of humans and the occurrence of cancer. Limited epidemiological data can be substantiated by evidence that the substance causes cancer by a mode of action that is relevant to man.

-2: Substances that are considered to be carcinogenic for man because sufficient data from long-term animal studies or limited evidence from animal studies substantiated by evidence from epidemiological studies indicate that they can make a significant contribution to cancer risk. Limited data from animal studies can be supported by evidence that the substance causes cancer by a mode of action that is relevant to man and by results of *in vitro* tests and short-term animal studies.

-3: Substances which cause concern that they could be carcinogenic for man but cannot be assessed conclusively because of lack of data. The classification in Category 3 is provisional.

-3A: Substances for which the criteria for classification in Category 4 or 5 are fulfilled but for which the database is insufficient for the establishment of a MAK value.

-3B: Substances for which *in vitro* tests or animal studies have yielded evidence of carcinogenic effects that is not sufficient for classification of the substance in one of the other categories. Further studies are required before a final classification can be made. A MAK or BAT value can be established, provided no genotoxic effects have been detected.

-4: Substances with carcinogenic potential for which genotoxicity plays no or at most a minor role. No significant contribution to human cancer risk is expected, provided the MAK value is observed. The classification is supported especially by evidence that increases in cellular proliferation or changes in cellular differentiation are important in the mode of action. To characterize the cancer risk, the manifold mechanisms contributing to carcinogenesis and their characteristic dose–time–response relationships are taken into consideration.

-5: Substances with carcinogenic and genotoxic effects, the potency of which is considered to be so low that, provided the MAK and BAT values are observed, no significant contribution to human cancer risk is to be expected. The classification is supported by information on the mode of action, dose-dependence, and toxicokinetic data pertinent to species comparison.

U.S. National Institute for Occupational Safety and Health (NIOSH)

NIOSH-Ca: Potential occupational carcinogen, with no further categorization.

U.S. National Toxicology Program (NTP)

NTP-K: Known to Be a Human Carcinogen — There is sufficient evidence of carcinogenicity from studies in humans which indicates a causal relationship between exposure to the agent, substance or mixture and human cancer.

-R: Reasonably Anticipated to Be a Human Carcinogen (RAHC) — There is limited evidence of carcinogenicity from studies in humans, which indicates that causal interpretation is credible, but that alternative explanations, such as chance, bias or confounding factors, could not adequately be excluded;

OR

There is sufficient evidence of carcinogenicity from studies in experimental animals which indicates there is an increased incidence of malignant and/or a combination of malignant and benign tumors: (1) in multiple species or at multiple tissue sites, or (2) by multiple routes of exposure, or (3) to an unusual degree with regard to incidence, site or type of tumor, or age at onset;

OR

There is less than sufficient evidence of carcinogenicity in humans or laboratory animals, however; the agent, substance or mixture belongs to a well defined, structurally-related class of substances whose members are listed in a previous Report on Carcinogens as either a known to be human carcinogen or reasonably anticipated to be human carcinogen, or there is convincing relevant information that the agent acts through mechanisms indicating it would likely cause cancer in humans.

U.S. Occupational Safety and Health Administration (OSHA)

OSHA-Ca: Carcinogen defined with no further categorization.

American Conference of Governmental Industrial Hygienists (ACGIH®)

TLV-A1: Confirmed Human Carcinogen — The agent is carcinogenic to humans based on the weight of evidence from epidemiologic studies.

-A2: Suspected Human Carcinogen — Human data are accepted as adequate in quality but are conflicting or insufficient to classify the agent as a confirmed human carcinogen; OR, the agent is carcinogenic in experimental animals at dose(s), by route(s) of exposure, at site(s), of histologic type(s), or by mechanism(s) considered relevant to worker exposure. The A2 is used primarily when there is limited evidence of carcinogenicity in humans and sufficient evidence of carcinogenicity in experimental animals with relevance to humans.

-A3: Confirmed Animal Carcinogen with Unknown Relevance to Humans — The agent is carcinogenic in experimental animals at a relatively high dose, by route(s) of administration, at site(s), of histologic type(s), or by mechanism(s) that may not be relevant to worker exposure. Available epidemiologic studies do not confirm an increased risk of cancer in exposed humans. Available evidence does not suggest that the agent is likely to cause cancer in humans except under uncommon or unlikely routes or levels of exposure.

-A4: Not Classifiable as a Human Carcinogen — Agents which cause concern that they could be carcinogenic for humans but which cannot be assessed conclusively because of a lack of data. In vitro or animal studies do not provide indications of carcinogenicity which are sufficient to classify the agent into one of the other categories.

-A5: Not Suspected as a Human Carcinogen — The agent is not suspected to be a human carcinogen on the basis of properly conducted epidemiologic studies in humans. These studies have sufficiently long follow-up, reliable exposure histories, sufficiently high dose, and adequate statistical power to conclude that exposure to the agent does not convey a significant risk of cancer to humans; OR, the evidence suggesting a lack of carcinogenicity in experimental animals is supported by mechanistic data.

Substances for which no human or experimental animal carcinogenic data have been reported are assigned no carcinogen designation.

Exposures to carcinogens must be kept to a minimum. Workers exposed to A1 carcinogens without a TLV® should be properly equipped to eliminate to the fullest extent possible all exposure to the carcinogen. For A1 carcinogens with a TLV® and for A2 and A3 carcinogens, worker exposure by all routes should be carefully controlled to levels as low as possible below the TLV®.

Notations

A-D listed in DFG MAK column only refers to Pregnancy Risk Group Classifications; see page xv for definitions.

(D) "Inert" gas or vapor that acts primarily as a simple asphyxiant without other significant physiologic effects when present in high concentrations in air.

DSEN May cause dermal sensitization. This notation is used to indicate the potential for dermal sensitization resulting from the interaction of an absorbed agent and ultraviolet light (i.e., photosensitization).

DSEN TLV Potential for worker sensitization by dermal contact as confirmed by available human or animal data.

E The value is for particulate matter containing no asbestos and < 1% Crystalline silica.

(F) Respirable fibers: length > 5 μ; aspect ratio ≥ 3:1, as determined by the membrane filter method at 400–450x magnification (4-mm objective), using phase-contrast illumination.

G As measured by the vertical elutriator, cotton-dust sampler. See Cotton Dust TLV® Documentation.

(H) Aerosol only.

I Measured as Inhalable fraction of the aerosol.

IFV Measured as Inhalable fraction and vapor.

(J) Does not include stearates of toxic metals.

(K) Should not exceed 2 mg/m³ respirable particulate.

L Exposure to carcinogens must be kept to a minimum. Workers exposed to A1 carcinogens without a TLV® should be properly equipped to eliminate to the fullest extent possible all exposure to the carcinogen. For A2 and A3 carcinogens without a TLV®, worker exposure by all routes should be carefully controlled. See the ACGIH® carcinogen definitions starting on the previous page.

(O) Sampled by method that does not collect vapor.

P Avoid prolonged and repeated skin contact to diesel fuels which can lead to dermal irritation and may be associated with an increased risk of skin cancer.

Q Absorbed rapidly through the skin in molten or heated liquid form in amounts that have caused rapid death in humans.

R Measured as respirable fraction of the aerosol.

RSEN May cause respiratory sensitization.

RSEN TLV Potential for worker sensitization by inhalation exposure as confirmed by available human or animal data.

Sa MAK–danger of sensitization of the airways.

SEN TLV–confirmed potential for worker sensitization as a result of dermal contact and/or inhalation exposure, based on the weight of scientific evidence.

Sh MAK–danger of sensitization of the skin.

Sah MAK–danger of sensitization of the airways and the skin.

SP MAK–danger of photo-contact sensitization.

T Measured as thoracic fraction of the aerosol.

(V) Vapor and aerosol.

(W) Worker exposure by all routes should be minimized to the fullest extent possible.

1-5 listed in the DFG MAK column only refers to Germ Cell Mutagen classifications; see page xv for definitions.

Miscellaneous

ACGIH® – American Conference of Governmental Industrial Hygienists

ACGIH® TLVs® – ACGIH® Threshold Limit Values

AIHA – American Industrial Hygiene Association

AIHA WEELs – AIHA Workplace Environmental Exposure Levels

BEI – ACGIH® has recommended a Biological Exposure Index or Indices (BEIs®) for this substance:
BEI$_A$ = Acetylcholinesterase Inhibiting Pesticides;
BEI$_M$ = Methemoglobin Inducers; and
BEI$_P$ = Polycyclic Aromatic Hydrocarbons (PAHs)
all of which are contained in the BEI® section of the current *TLVs®* and *BEIs®* Book. For proper application, read the *BEI® Documentation* for the substance.

CAS – Chemical Abstracts Service Registry Number

Ceiling (C) – The concentration that shall not be exceeded during any part of the working exposure

MAK – Federal Republic of Germany Maximum Concentration Values at the Workplace

NIC – Notice of Intended Changes

NIOSH Ceiling – The exposure that shall not be exceeded during any part of the workday. If instantaneous monitoring is not feasible, the ceiling shall be assessed as a 15-minute TWA exposure (unless otherwise specified) that shall not be exceeded at any time during a workday.

NIOSH RELs – U.S. National Institute for Occupational Safety and Health Recommended Exposure Limits. For NIOSH RELs, TWA indicates a time-weighted average concentration for up to a 10-hour workday during a 40-hour workweek.

OSHA PELs – U.S. Occupational Safety and Health Administration Permissible Exposure Limits

Skin – Danger of cutaneous absorption

STEL – Short-Term Exposure Limit. Usually a 15-minute time-weighted average (TWA) exposure that should not be exceeded at any time during a workday, even if the 8-hour TWA is within the TLV–TWA, PEL–TWA, or REL–TWA

TWA – Time-weighted average exposure concentration for a conventional 8-hour (TLV®, PEL) or up to a 10-hour (REL) workday and a 40-hour workweek

( ) – Values/notations contained in parentheses under the ACGIH® TLV® column indicate that these are under review and that an NIC exists.

MAK EXCURSION FACTORS, MAXIMUM DURATION OF PEAKS, MAXIMUM NUMBER PER SHIFT, AND MINIMUM INTERVAL BETWEEN PEAKS

Category	Excursion Factor	Duration	Number per Shift	Interval[A]
I Substances for which local Irritant effects determine the MAK value, also respiratory allergens	1[B]	15 min, average value[C]	4	1 hour
II Substances with systemic effects	2[B]	15 min, average value	4	1 hour

[A] Only for excursion factors > 1.

[B] Default value, or a substance-specific value (maximum 8).

[C] In certain cases, a momentary value (concentration that should not be exceeded at any time) can also be established.

MAK PREGNANCY RISK GROUP CLASSIFICATION

Group A: Damage to the embryo or foetus in humans has been unequivocally demonstrated and is to be expected even when MAK and BAT values are observed.

Group B: According to currently available information, damage to the embryo or foetus must be expected even when MAK and BAT values are observed.

Group C: There is no reason to fear damage to the embryo or foetus when MAK and BAT values are observed.

Group D: Either there are no data for an assessment of damage to the embryo or foetus or the currently available data are not sufficient for classification in one of the groups A–C.

MAK GERM CELL MUTAGENS (confirmed or suspected)*

1. Germ cell mutagens which have been shown to increase the mutant frequency in the progeny of exposed humans.
2. Germ cell mutagens which have been shown to increase the mutant frequency in the progeny of exposed mammals.
3A. Substances which have been shown to induce genetic damage in germ cells of humans or animals, or which produce mutagenic effects in somatic cells of mammals *in vivo* and have been shown to reach the germ cells in an active form.
3B. Substances which are suspected of being germ cell mutagens because of their genotoxic effects in mammalian somatic cells *in vivo*; in exceptional cases, substances for which there are no *in vivo* data but which are clearly mutagenic *in vitro* and structurally related to known *in vivo* mutagens.
4. Not applicable. (Category 4 carcinogenic substances are those with nongenotoxic mechanisms of action. By definition, germ cell mutagens are genotoxic. Therefore, a Category 4 for germ cell mutagens cannot apply. At some time in the future, it is conceivable that a Category 4 could be established for genotoxic substances with primary targets other than DNA [e.g., purely aneugenic substances] if research results make this seem sensible.)
5. Germ cell mutagens or suspected substances (according to the definition of Category 3A and 3B), the potency of which is considered to be so low that, provided the MAK value is observed, their contribution to genetic risk for humans is expected not to be significant.

*The Categories for classification of germ cell mutagens have been established by analogy with the categories for carcinogenic chemicals at the workplace.

| SUBSTANCE | ACGIH® TLVs® | | | | OSHA PELs | | | | NIOSH RELs | | | | DFG MAKs | | | | AIHA WEELs | | | | CARCINOGENICITY |
| | TWA | | STEL/CEIL(C) | | TWA | | STEL/CEIL(C) | | TWA | | STEL/CEIL(C) | | TWA | | PEAK/CEIL(C) | | TWA | | STEL/CEIL(C) | | |
CAS#	ppm	mg/m³	ppm	mg/m³	ppm	mg/m³	ppm	mg/m³	ppm	mg/m³	ppm	mg/m³	ppm	mg/m³	ppm	mg/m³	ppm	mg/m³	ppm	mg/m³	CATEGORY
Abietic acid 514-10-3														Sh							
Acenaphthene 83-32-9																					IARC-3
Acenaphthylene 208-96-8																					EPA-D
Acephate 30560-19-1																					EPA-C
Acepyrene 25732-74-5																					IARC-3
Acetaldehyde (Acetic aldehyde) 75-07-0			C 25	C 45	200	360							50	91	I (1) C 100 C 180 C; 5						EPA-B2 NTP-R IARC-2B (TLV-A3) MAK-5 NIOSH-Ca
			NIC-A2						*See* Pocket Guide Apps. A and C												
Acetamide 60-35-5																					IARC-2B MAK-3B
Acetaminophen (Paracetamol) 103-90-2																					IARC-3
Acetic acid 64-19-7	10	25	15	37	10	25			10	25	15	37	10	25	I (2) C						

SUBSTANCE / CAS#	ACGIH® TLVs® TWA ppm	TWA mg/m³	STEL/CEIL(C) ppm	STEL/CEIL(C) mg/m³	OSHA PELs TWA ppm	TWA mg/m³	STEL/CEIL(C) ppm	STEL/CEIL(C) mg/m³	NIOSH RELs TWA ppm	TWA mg/m³	STEL/CEIL(C) ppm	STEL/CEIL(C) mg/m³	DFG MAKs TWA ppm	TWA mg/m³	PEAK/CEIL(C) ppm	PEAK/CEIL(C) mg/m³	AIHA WEELs TWA ppm	TWA mg/m³	STEL/CEIL(C) ppm	STEL/CEIL(C) mg/m³	CARCINOGENICITY CATEGORY
Acetic anhydride 108-24-7	1	4	C 3		5	20					C 5	C 20	5	21	I (1) D						TLV-A4
Acetone 67-64-1	(500) NIC-200	(1188) NIC-475	(750) NIC-500 BEI	(1782) NIC-1187	1000	2400			250	590			500	1200	I (2) B						EPA-I (TLV-A4)
Acetone cyanohydrin 75-86-5			C 5* *as CN Skin								C 1* *15-min	C 4*					2		5 Skin		
Acetonitrile 75-05-8	20	34 Skin			40	70			20	34			20	34 Skin; C	II (2)						EPA-CBD; D TLV-A4
Acetophenone 98-86-2	10	49															10				EPA-D
2-Acetylaminofluorene (2-AAF) 53-96-3					*See* 29 CFR 1910.1014				*See* Pocket Guide App. A												NIOSH-Ca NTP-R OSHA-Ca
Acetyl chloride 75-36-5																					EPA-D
Acetylene 74-86-2		Simple asphyxiant(D)									C 2500	C 2662									
Acetylsalicylic acid (Aspirin) 50-78-2		5								5											

SUBSTANCE / CAS#	ACGIH® TLVs® TWA ppm	mg/m³	STEL/CEIL(C) ppm	mg/m³	OSHA PELs TWA ppm	mg/m³	STEL/CEIL(C) ppm	mg/m³	NIOSH RELs TWA ppm	mg/m³	STEL/CEIL(C) ppm	mg/m³	DFG MAKs TWA ppm	mg/m³	PEAK/CEIL(C) ppm	mg/m³	AIHA WEELs TWA ppm	mg/m³	STEL/CEIL(C) ppm	mg/m³	CARCINOGENICITY CATEGORY
Aciclovir 59277-89-3																					IARC-3
Acridine Orange 494-38-2																					IARC-3
Acriflavinium chloride 8018-07-3																					IARC-3
Acrolein 107-02-8			C 0.1	C 0.23	0.1	0.25			0.1	0.25	0.3	0.8									EPA-I IARC-3 MAK-3B TLV-A4
	Skin								*See* Pocket Guide App. C												
Acrylamide 79-06-1	0.03 **IFV**				0.3				0.03												EPA-L IARC-2A MAK-2 NIOSH-Ca NTP-R TLV-A3
	Skin				Skin				Skin *See* Pocket Guide App. A				Skin; Sh; 2								
Acrylic acid 79-10-7	2	5.9							2	6			10	30	I (1)						IARC-3 TLV-A4
	Skin								Skin				C								
Acrylic acid polymer, neutralized, cross-linked 9003-04-7													0.05 **R**		I (1)						MAK-4
													C								
Acrylonitrile (Vinyl cyanide) 107-13-1	2	4.3			2		C 10		1		C 10*										EPA-B1 IARC-2B MAK-2 NIOSH-Ca NTP-R OSHA-Ca TLV-A3
	Skin				Skin *See* 29 CFR 1910.1045				Skin *15-min *See* Pocket Guide App. A				Skin; Sh								
Actinomycin D 50-76-0																					IARC-3

SUBSTANCE / CAS#	ACGIH® TLVs® TWA ppm	TWA mg/m³	STEL/CEIL(C) ppm	STEL/CEIL(C) mg/m³	OSHA PELs TWA ppm	TWA mg/m³	STEL/CEIL(C) ppm	STEL/CEIL(C) mg/m³	NIOSH RELs TWA ppm	TWA mg/m³	STEL/CEIL(C) ppm	STEL/CEIL(C) mg/m³	DFG MAKs TWA ppm	TWA mg/m³	PEAK/CEIL(C) ppm	PEAK/CEIL(C) mg/m³	AIHA WEELs TWA ppm	TWA mg/m³	STEL/CEIL(C) ppm	STEL/CEIL(C) mg/m³	CARCINOGENICITY CATEGORY
Adipic acid 124-04-9		5																			
Adiponitrile 111-69-3	2	8.8							4	18											EPA-D
	Skin																				
Adriamycin®, Doxorubicin hydrochloride 23214-92-8																					IARC-2A NTP-R
Aflatoxins 1402-68-2														Skin; 3A							IARC-1; 2B* MAK-1 NTP-K *CAS: 6795-23-9
Agaritine 2757-90-6																					IARC-3
Alachlor 15972-60-8		1 IFV																			TLV-A3
	(SEN) NIC-DSEN																				
Aldicarb 116-06-3																		0.0001			EPA-D IARC-3
																		Skin			
Aldrin 309-00-2		0.05 IFV				0.25				0.25				0.25 I		II (8)					EPA-B2 IARC-3 NIOSH-Ca TLV-A3
	Skin				Skin				Skin *See* Pocket Guide App. A				Skin							

SUBSTANCE / CAS#	ACGIH® TLVs® TWA ppm	mg/m³	STEL/CEIL(C) ppm	mg/m³	OSHA PELs TWA ppm	mg/m³	STEL/CEIL(C) ppm	mg/m³	NIOSH RELs TWA ppm	mg/m³	STEL/CEIL(C) ppm	mg/m³	DFG MAKs TWA ppm	mg/m³	PEAK/CEIL(C) ppm	mg/m³	AIHA WEELs TWA ppm	mg/m³	STEL/CEIL(C) ppm	mg/m³	CARCINOGENICITY CATEGORY
Aliphatic hydrocarbon gases, Alkanes [C$_1$-C$_4$]	TLV® withdrawn. Methane, Ethane, Propane, Liquefied petroleum gas (LPG) and Natural gas – refer to Appendix F: Minimal Oxygen Content. Butane and Isobutane – refer to Butane, all isomers																				
Alkali persulfates													Sah								
Allyl alcohol (AA) 107-18-6	0.5	1.19			2	5			2	5	4	10									MAK-3B TLV-A4
	Skin				Skin				Skin				Skin								
Allyl bromide 106-95-6	0.1	0.5	0.2	1.0																	TLV-A4
	Skin																				
Allyl chloride 107-05-1	1	3	2	6	1	3			1	3	2	6									EPA-C IARC-3 MAK-3B TLV-A3
	Skin												Skin								
Allyl glycidyl ether (AGE) 106-92-3	1	4.7					C 10	C 45	5	22	10	44									MAK-2 TLV-A4
									Skin				Skin; Sh								
Allyl isothiocyanate 57-06-7																				1	IARC-3
																Skin; DSEN				
Allyl isovalerate 2835-39-4																					IARC-3

SUBSTANCE / CAS#	ACGIH® TLVs® TWA ppm	mg/m³	STEL/CEIL(C) ppm	mg/m³	OSHA PELs TWA ppm	mg/m³	STEL/CEIL(C) ppm	mg/m³	NIOSH RELs TWA ppm	mg/m³	STEL/CEIL(C) ppm	mg/m³	DFG MAKs TWA ppm	mg/m³	PEAK/CEIL(C) ppm	mg/m³	AIHA WEELs TWA ppm	mg/m³	STEL/CEIL(C) ppm	mg/m³	CARCINOGENICITY CATEGORY
Allyl propyl disulfide 2179-59-1	0.5	3			2	12			2	12	3	18	2	12	I (1)						
	(SEN) NIC-DSEN																				
Aluminum hydroxide 21645-51-2														4 I 1.5 R D							
Aluminum oxide (α-Alumina) 1344-28-1	TLV® withdrawn; *see* Aluminum, metal and insoluble compounds				15*; 5** *Total dust **Respirable fraction									4 I 1.5 R D							MAK-2* *Fibrous dust
Aluminum, alkyls, not otherwise specified, as Al	TLV® withdrawn; *see* Aluminum, metal and insoluble compounds									2											
Aluminum, metal and insoluble compounds 7429-90-5	1 R				15*; 5** *Total dust **Respirable fraction				10*; 5** *Total dust **Respirable fraction					4 I 1.5 R D							IARC-1* TLV-A4 *production
Aluminum, pyro powders and welding fumes, as Al	TLV® withdrawn for Welding fumes as a result of Appendix B removal									5											
Aluminum, soluble salts and alkyls, as Al	TLV® withdrawn; *see* Aluminum, metal and insoluble compounds									2											
Amaranth 915-67-3																					IARC-3
5-Aminoacenaphthene 4657-93-6																					IARC-3

SUBSTANCE CAS#	ACGIH® TLVs® TWA ppm	mg/m³	STEL/CEIL(C) ppm	mg/m³	OSHA PELs TWA ppm	mg/m³	STEL/CEIL(C) ppm	mg/m³	NIOSH RELs TWA ppm	mg/m³	STEL/CEIL(C) ppm	mg/m³	DFG MAKs TWA ppm	mg/m³	PEAK/CEIL(C) ppm	mg/m³	AIHA WEELs TWA ppm	mg/m³	STEL/CEIL(C) ppm	mg/m³	CARCINOGENICITY CATEGORY
2-Aminoanthraquinone 117-79-3																					IARC-3 NTP-R
p-Aminoazobenzene 60-09-3													Sh								IARC-2B
o-Aminoazotoluene 97-56-3													Skin; Sh; 3B								IARC-2B MAK-2 NTP-R
p-Aminobenzoic acid 150-13-0																		5			IARC-3
1-Amino-2,4-dibromo-anthraquinone 81-49-2																					IARC-2B NTP-R
2-Amino-3,4-dimethyl-imidazo[4,5-f]quinoline (MeIQ) 77094-11-2																					IARC-2B NTP-R
2-Amino-3,8-dimethyl-imidazo[4,5-f]quinoxaline (MeIQx) 77500-04-0																					IARC-2B NTP-R
3-Amino-1,4-dimethyl-5H-pyrido[4,3-b]indole (Trp-P-1) 62450-06-0																					IARC-2B
4-Aminodiphenyl 92-67-1	Skin; L				See 29 CFR 1910.1003				See Pocket Guide App. A				Skin								IARC-1 OSHA-Ca MAK-1 TLV-A1 NIOSH-Ca NTP-K

SUBSTANCE / CAS#	ACGIH® TLVs® TWA ppm	mg/m³	STEL/CEIL(C) ppm	mg/m³	OSHA PELs TWA ppm	mg/m³	STEL/CEIL(C) ppm	mg/m³	NIOSH RELs TWA ppm	mg/m³	STEL/CEIL(C) ppm	mg/m³	DFG MAKs TWA ppm	mg/m³	PEAK/CEIL(C) ppm	mg/m³	AIHA WEELs TWA ppm	mg/m³	STEL/CEIL(C) ppm	mg/m³	CARCINOGENICITY CATEGORY
4-Aminodiphenylamine 101-54-2													Skin; Sh; 3B								
2-Aminodipyrido[1,2-a: 3′,2′-d]imidazole (Glu-P-2) 67730-10-3																					IARC-2B
6-Amino-2-ethoxy-naphthalene 293733-21-8																					MAK-2
3-Amino-9-ethyl-carbazole 132-32-1																					MAK-3B
1-Amino-2-methyl-anthraquinone 82-28-0																					IARC-3 NTP-R
2-Amino-6-methyldipyri-do[1,2-a:3′,2′-d]imida-zole (Glu-P-1) 67730-11-4																					IARC-2B
2-Amino-3-methylimid-azo[4,5-f]quinoline (IQ) 76180-96-6																					IARC-2A NTP-R
2-Amino-1-methyl-6-phe-nylimidazo[4,5-b]pyridine (PhIP) 105650-23-5																					IARC-2B NTP-R
3-Amino-1-methyl-5H-pyrido[4,3-b]indole (Trp-P-2) 62450-07-1																					IARC-2B

SUBSTANCE / CAS#	ACGIH® TLVs® TWA ppm	mg/m³	STEL/CEIL(C) ppm	mg/m³	OSHA PELs TWA ppm	mg/m³	STEL/CEIL(C) ppm	mg/m³	NIOSH RELs TWA ppm	mg/m³	STEL/CEIL(C) ppm	mg/m³	DFG MAKs TWA ppm	mg/m³	PEAK/CEIL(C) ppm	mg/m³	AIHA WEELs TWA ppm	mg/m³	STEL/CEIL(C) ppm	mg/m³	CARCINOGENICITY CATEGORY
2-Amino-3-methyl-9H-pyrido[2,3-b]indole (MeA-α-C) 68006-83-7																					IARC-2B
3-Aminomethyl-3,5,5-trimethyl cyclohexylamine (Isophorone diamine) 2855-13-2														Sh							
2-Amino-5-(5-nitro-2-furyl)-1,3,4-thiadiazole 712-68-5																					IARC-2B
2-Amino-4-nitrophenol 99-57-0																					IARC-3
2-Amino-5-nitrophenol 121-88-0																					IARC-3
2-Amino-5-nitrothiazole 121-66-4																					IARC-3
p-Aminophenol 123-30-8														Sh							
3-Aminophenyl 591-27-5														Sh							
bis(4-Aminophenyl) ether (4,4'-Oxydianiline; 4,4'-Diaminodiphenyl) 101-80-4																					IARC-2B MAK-2 NTP-R

SUBSTANCE / CAS#	ACGIH® TLVs® TWA ppm	mg/m³	STEL/CEIL(C) ppm	mg/m³	OSHA PELs TWA ppm	mg/m³	STEL/CEIL(C) ppm	mg/m³	NIOSH RELs TWA ppm	mg/m³	STEL/CEIL(C) ppm	mg/m³	DFG MAKs TWA ppm	mg/m³	PEAK/CEIL(C) ppm	mg/m³	AIHA WEELs TWA ppm	mg/m³	STEL/CEIL(C) ppm	mg/m³	CARCINOGENICITY CATEGORY
2-Aminopyridine 504-29-0	0.5	2			0.5	2			0.5	2											
4-Aminopyridine 504-24-5																					EPA-D
2-Amino-9H-pyrido [2,3-b]indole (A-α-C) 26148-68-5																					IARC-2B
Aminotris(methylene-phosphonic acid) 6419-19-8																	10				
11-Aminoundecanoic acid 2432-99-7																					IARC-3
Amitrole (3-Amino-1,2,4-triazole) 61-82-5		0.2								0.2				0.2 I	II (8)						IARC-3 TLV-A3 MAK-4 NIOSH-Ca NTP-R
									See Pocket Guide App. A				Skin; C								
Ammonia 7664-41-7	25	17	35	24	50	35			25	18	35	27	20	14	I (2) C						
Ammonium acetate 631-61-8																					EPA-D
Ammonium chloride fume 12125-02-9		10		20						10		20									

SUBSTANCE CAS#	ACGIH® TLVs® TWA ppm	ACGIH® TLVs® TWA mg/m³	ACGIH® TLVs® STEL/CEIL(C) ppm	ACGIH® TLVs® STEL/CEIL(C) mg/m³	OSHA PELs TWA ppm	OSHA PELs TWA mg/m³	OSHA PELs STEL/CEIL(C) ppm	OSHA PELs STEL/CEIL(C) mg/m³	NIOSH RELs TWA ppm	NIOSH RELs TWA mg/m³	NIOSH RELs STEL/CEIL(C) ppm	NIOSH RELs STEL/CEIL(C) mg/m³	DFG MAKs TWA ppm	DFG MAKs TWA mg/m³	DFG MAKs PEAK/CEIL(C) ppm	DFG MAKs PEAK/CEIL(C) mg/m³	AIHA WEELs TWA ppm	AIHA WEELs TWA mg/m³	AIHA WEELs STEL/CEIL(C) ppm	AIHA WEELs STEL/CEIL(C) mg/m³	CARCINOGENICITY CATEGORY
Ammonium methacrylate 16325-47-6																					EPA-D
Ammonium perfluorooctanoate 3825-26-1		0.01 Skin																			TLV-A3
Ammonium persulfate, as S_2O_8 7727-54-0		0.1												Sah							
Ammonium sulfamate 7773-06-0		10			15*; 5**		*Total dust **Respirable fraction		10*; 5**		*Total dust **Respirable fraction										
Amsacrine 51264-14-3																					IARC-2B
α-Amylase														Sa							
α-Amylcinnamalde-hyde 122-40-7														Sh							
tert-Amyl methyl ether (TAME) 994-05-8	20	84																			
Angelicin plus ultra-violet A radiation 523-50-2																					IARC-3

SUBSTANCE	ACGIH® TLVs®				OSHA PELs				NIOSH RELs				DFG MAKs				AIHA WEELs				CARCINOGENICITY CATEGORY
	TWA		STEL/CEIL(C)		TWA		STEL/CEIL(C)		TWA		STEL/CEIL(C)		TWA		PEAK/CEIL(C)		TWA		STEL/CEIL(C)		
CAS#	ppm	mg/m³	ppm	mg/m³	ppm	mg/m³	ppm	mg/m³	ppm	mg/m³	ppm	mg/m³	ppm	mg/m³	ppm	mg/m³	ppm	mg/m³	ppm	mg/m³	
Aniline 62-53-3	2	7.6 Skin; BEI			5	19 and Homologues Skin			and Homologues See Pocket Guide App. A				2	7.7 Skin; Sh; C	II (2)						EPA-B2 TLV-A3 IARC-3 MAK-4 NIOSH-Ca
Animal hair, epithelia and other materials derived from animals														Sah							
Anisidine, o-isomer 90-04-0	0.1	0.5 Skin; BEI_M				0.5 Skin				0.5 Skin See Pocket Guide App. A				Skin							IARC-2B MAK-2 NIOSH-Ca TLV-A3
Anisidine, p-isomer 104-94-9	0.1	0.5 Skin; BEI_M				0.5 Skin				0.5 Skin				Skin							IARC-3 MAK-3B TLV-A4
Anisidine hydrochloride, o-isomer 134-29-2																					NTP-R
Anthanthrene 191-26-4														Skin							IARC-3 MAK-2
Anthracene 120-12-7																					EPA-D IARC-3
Anthranilic acid 118-92-3																					IARC-3
Anthraquinone 84-65-1																					IARC-2B

SUBSTANCE / CAS#	ACGIH® TLVs® TWA ppm	mg/m³	STEL/CEIL(C) ppm	mg/m³	OSHA PELs TWA ppm	mg/m³	STEL/CEIL(C) ppm	mg/m³	NIOSH RELs TWA ppm	mg/m³	STEL/CEIL(C) ppm	mg/m³	DFG MAKs TWA ppm	mg/m³	PEAK/CEIL(C) ppm	mg/m³	AIHA WEELs TWA ppm	mg/m³	STEL/CEIL(C) ppm	mg/m³	CARCINOGENICITY CATEGORY
Antimony [7440-36-0] and compounds, as Sb		0.5				0.5				0.5			and inorganic compounds excluding Stibine 3B								MAK-2
Antimony hydride (Stibine) 7803-52-3	0.1	0.51			0.1	0.5			0.1	0.5											
Antimony oxide 1327-33-9													3B								MAK-2
Antimony trioxide, as Sb 1309-64-4		0.5				0.5				0.5			3B								IARC-2B MAK-2
Antimony trioxide production 1309-64-4		L																			TLV-A2
Antimony trisulfide 1345-04-6																					IARC-3
ANTU (α-Naphthylthiourea) 86-88-4		0.3 Skin				0.3				0.3			Skin								IARC-3 MAK-3B TLV-A4
Apholate 52-46-0																					IARC-3
Apollo 74115-24-5																					EPA-C

SUBSTANCE / CAS#	ACGIH® TLVs®				OSHA PELs				NIOSH RELs				DFG MAKs				AIHA WEELs				CARCINOGENICITY CATEGORY
	TWA		STEL/CEIL(C)		TWA		STEL/CEIL(C)		TWA		STEL/CEIL(C)		TWA		PEAK/CEIL(C)		TWA		STEL/CEIL(C)		
	ppm	mg/m³	ppm	mg/m³	ppm	mg/m³	ppm	mg/m³	ppm	mg/m³	ppm	mg/m³	ppm	mg/m³	ppm	mg/m³	ppm	mg/m³	ppm	mg/m³	
p–Aramide, fibrous dust 26125-61-1																					MAK-3B
Aramite® 140-57-8																					EPA-B2 IARC-2B
Argon 7440-37-1	NIC-withdraw TLV®; refer to Appendix F: Minimal Oxygen Content (Simple asphyxiant(D))																				
Aristolochic acid 313-67-7																					IARC-1 NTP-K
Arsenic [7440-38-2] and inorganic compounds (except arsine), as As	0.01	BEI			0.5**; 0.01* **Organic compounds *Inorganic compounds 29 CFR 1910.1018 Inorgan. cpds.						C 0.002* *15-min See Pocket Guide App. A			3A							EPA-A IARC-1 MAK-1 NIOSH-Ca NTP-K OSHA-Ca TLV-A1
Arsenic acid [7778-39-4] and its salts, as As	0.01													3A							EPA-A IARC-1 MAK-1 NIOSH-Ca NTP-K OSHA-Ca TLV-A1
Arsenic pentoxide, as As 1303-28-2	0.01													3A							MAK-1 TLV-A1
Arsenic trioxide, as As 1327-53-3	0.01													3A							MAK-1 TLV-A1

SUBSTANCE CAS#	ACGIH® TLVs® TWA ppm	mg/m³	STEL/CEIL(C) ppm	mg/m³	OSHA PELs TWA ppm	mg/m³	STEL/CEIL(C) ppm	mg/m³	NIOSH RELs TWA ppm	mg/m³	STEL/CEIL(C) ppm	mg/m³	DFG MAKs TWA ppm	mg/m³	PEAK/CEIL(C) ppm	mg/m³	AIHA WEELs TWA ppm	mg/m³	STEL/CEIL(C) ppm	mg/m³	CARCINOGENICITY CATEGORY
Arsenous [13464-58-9] **acid and its salts, as As**		0.01												3A							EPA-A NTP-K IARC-1 OSHA-Ca MAK-1 TLV-A1 NIOSH-Ca
Arsine 7784-42-1	0.005	0.01			0.05	0.2					C 0.002* *15-min See Pocket Guide App. A										NIOSH-Ca
Asbestos, all forms 1332-21-4; 12001-28-4; 12172-73-5; 77536-66-4; 77536-67-5; 77536-68-6; 132207-32-0		0.1 f/cc(F)			0.1 f/cc	1 f/cc* *30-min See 29 CFR 1910.1001			See Pocket Guide Apps. A and C												EPA-A IARC-1 MAK-1 NIOSH-Ca NTP-K OSHA-Ca TLV-A1
Asphalt fume (Bitumen) 8052-42-4		0.5 I as benzene-soluble aerosol BEI_P									C 5* *15-min See Pocket Guide App. A			Skin; (V)							IARC-2B*; 2A** NIOSH-Ca MAK-2 TLV-A4 * hard bitumens and emissions during mastic asphalt work; straight run bitumens emissions during road paving ** oxidized bitumens emissions during roofing
Assure 76578-14-8																					EPA-D
Atrazine 1912-24-9		(5) NIC-2 I NIC-A3								5				1 I C		II (2)					IARC-3 (TLV-A4)
Attapulgite, fibrous dust (Palygorskite) 12174-11-7																					IARC-2B*; 3** MAK-2 *> 5 μm **< 5 μm

SUBSTANCE / CAS#	ACGIH® TLVs® TWA ppm	ACGIH® TLVs® TWA mg/m³	ACGIH® TLVs® STEL/CEIL(C) ppm	ACGIH® TLVs® STEL/CEIL(C) mg/m³	OSHA PELs TWA ppm	OSHA PELs TWA mg/m³	OSHA PELs STEL/CEIL(C) ppm	OSHA PELs STEL/CEIL(C) mg/m³	NIOSH RELs TWA ppm	NIOSH RELs TWA mg/m³	NIOSH RELs STEL/CEIL(C) ppm	NIOSH RELs STEL/CEIL(C) mg/m³	DFG MAKs TWA ppm	DFG MAKs TWA mg/m³	DFG MAKs PEAK/CEIL(C) ppm	DFG MAKs PEAK/CEIL(C) mg/m³	AIHA WEELs TWA ppm	AIHA WEELs TWA mg/m³	AIHA WEELs STEL/CEIL(C) ppm	AIHA WEELs STEL/CEIL(C) mg/m³	CARCINOGENICITY CATEGORY
Auramine 492-80-8														Skin; 3B							IARC-1*; 2B MAK-2 *production
Auramine hydrochloride 2465-27-2														Skin; 3B							MAK-2
Aurothioglucose 12192-57-3																					IARC-3
Azacitidine 320-67-2																					IARC-2A NTP-R
Azaserine 115-02-6																					IARC-2B
Azathioprine 446-86-6																					IARC-1 NTP-K
Azinphos-methyl 86-50-0		0.2 **IFV** Skin; (SEN); BEI_A NIC-DSEN				0.2 Skin				0.2 Skin				0.2 **I** Skin	II (8)						TLV-A4
tris(Aziridinyl)-p-benzo-quinone (Triaziquone) 68-76-8																					IARC-3
2-(1-Aziridinyl)ethanol 1072-52-2																					IARC-3

SUBSTANCE / CAS#	ACGIH® TLVs® TWA ppm	TWA mg/m³	STEL/CEIL(C) ppm	mg/m³	OSHA PELs TWA ppm	mg/m³	STEL/CEIL(C) ppm	mg/m³	NIOSH RELs TWA ppm	mg/m³	STEL/CEIL(C) ppm	mg/m³	DFG MAKs TWA ppm	mg/m³	PEAK/CEIL(C) ppm	mg/m³	AIHA WEELs TWA ppm	mg/m³	STEL/CEIL(C) ppm	mg/m³	CARCINOGENICITY CATEGORY
bis(1-Aziridinyl)morpholinophosphine sulfide (Morzid) 2168-68-5																					IARC-3
tris(1-Aziridinyl)-phosphine oxide 545-55-1																					IARC-3
2,4,6-tris(1-Aziridinyl)-s-triazine 51-18-3																					IARC-3
Aziridyl benzoquinone 800-24-8																					IARC-3
Azobenzene 103-33-3																					EPA-B2 IARC-3
Barium [7440-39-3] and soluble compounds, as Ba		0.5				0.5				0.5				0.5 I	II (8)						EPA-CBD*; NL**; D TLV-A4 *inhalation **oral
													Soluble compounds only D								
Barium sulfate 7727-43-7		(10) NIC-5 I				15*; 5**				10*; 5**				4 I 1.5 R C							
					*Total dust **Respirable fraction				*Total dust **Respirable fraction											
Benomyl 17804-35-2		1 I (SEN) NIC-DSEN				15*; 5**								Sh; 3A							TLV-A3
					*Total dust **Respirable fraction															
Bentazon (Basagran) 25057-89-0																					EPA-NL; E

SUBSTANCE / CAS#	ACGIH® TLVs® TWA ppm	TWA mg/m³	STEL/CEIL(C) ppm	STEL/CEIL(C) mg/m³	OSHA PELs TWA ppm	TWA mg/m³	STEL/CEIL(C) ppm	STEL/CEIL(C) mg/m³	NIOSH RELs TWA ppm	TWA mg/m³	STEL/CEIL(C) ppm	STEL/CEIL(C) mg/m³	DFG MAKs TWA ppm	TWA mg/m³	PEAK/CEIL(C) ppm	PEAK/CEIL(C) mg/m³	AIHA WEELs TWA ppm	TWA mg/m³	STEL/CEIL(C) ppm	STEL/CEIL(C) mg/m³	CARCINOGENICITY CATEGORY
11H-Benz[bc]aceanthrylene 202-94-8																					IARC-3
Benz[j]aceanthrylene 203-33-5																					IARC-2B
Benz[l]aceanthrylene 211-91-6																					IARC-3
Benz[a]acridine 225-11-6																					IARC-3
Benz[c]acridine 225-51-4																					IARC-3
Benzal chloride (Benzyl dichloride) 98-87-3														Skin							IARC-2A MAK-2
Benzaldehyde 100-52-7																	2		4		
																	DSEN				
Benz[a]anthracene 56-55-3		L; BEI_P												Skin; 3A							EPA-B2 TLV-A2 IARC-2B MAK-2 NTP-R
Benzene 71-43-2	0.5	1.6	2.5	8	1* Skin; BEI	3*	5*	15*	0.1		1			Skin; 3A							EPA-A; K NTP-K IARC-1 OSHA-Ca MAK-1 TLV-A1 NIOSH-Ca

*Table Z-2 for exclusions in 29 CFR 1910.1028(d)
See 29 CFR 1910.1028
See Pocket Guide App. A

SUBSTANCE / CAS#	ACGIH® TLVs® TWA ppm	mg/m³	STEL/CEIL(C) ppm	mg/m³	OSHA PELs TWA ppm	mg/m³	STEL/CEIL(C) ppm	mg/m³	NIOSH RELs TWA ppm	mg/m³	STEL/CEIL(C) ppm	mg/m³	DFG MAKs TWA ppm	mg/m³	PEAK/CEIL(C) ppm	mg/m³	AIHA WEELs TWA ppm	mg/m³	STEL/CEIL(C) ppm	mg/m³	CARCINOGENICITY CATEGORY
Benzidine 92-87-5	Skin; L				See 29 CFR 1910.1003				See Pocket Guide Apps. A and C				and its salts Skin								EPA-A NTP-K IARC-1* OSHA-Ca MAK-1 TLV-A1 NIOSH-Ca *including dyes metabolized to Benzidine
Benzidine-based dyes					minimize exposure; handle with caution See Pocket Guide App. C																NIOSH-Ca
1,2-Benzisothiazol-3(2H)-one 2634-33-5													Sh								
Benzo[b]chrysene 214-17-5																					IARC-3
Benzo[g]chrysene 196-78-1																					IARC-3
Benzo[a]fluoranthene 203-33-8																					IARC-3
Benzo[b]fluoranthene 205-99-2	L; BEI_P												Skin; 3B								EPA-B2 TLV-A2 IARC-2B MAK-2 NTP-R
Benzo[ghi]fluoranthene 203-12-3																					IARC-3
Benzo[j]fluoranthene 205-82-3													Skin; 3B								IARC-2B MAK-2 NTP-R

SUBSTANCE / CAS#	ACGIH® TLVs® TWA ppm	ACGIH® TLVs® TWA mg/m³	ACGIH® TLVs® STEL/CEIL(C) ppm	ACGIH® TLVs® STEL/CEIL(C) mg/m³	OSHA PELs TWA ppm	OSHA PELs TWA mg/m³	OSHA PELs STEL/CEIL(C) ppm	OSHA PELs STEL/CEIL(C) mg/m³	NIOSH RELs TWA ppm	NIOSH RELs TWA mg/m³	NIOSH RELs STEL/CEIL(C) ppm	NIOSH RELs STEL/CEIL(C) mg/m³	DFG MAKs TWA ppm	DFG MAKs TWA mg/m³	DFG MAKs PEAK/CEIL(C) ppm	DFG MAKs PEAK/CEIL(C) mg/m³	AIHA WEELs TWA ppm	AIHA WEELs TWA mg/m³	AIHA WEELs STEL/CEIL(C) ppm	AIHA WEELs STEL/CEIL(C) mg/m³	CARCINOGENICITY CATEGORY
Benzo[k]fluoranthene 207-08-9															Skin; 3B						EPA-B2 IARC-2B MAK-2 NTP-R
Benzo[a]fluorene 238-84-6																					IARC-3
Benzo[b]fluorene 243-17-4																					IARC-3
Benzo[c]fluorene 205-12-9																					IARC-3
Benzofuran 271-89-6																					IARC-2B
Benzoic acid 65-85-0																					EPA-D
Benzo[b]naphtho-[2,1-d]-thiophene 239-35-0															Skin; 3B						IARC-3 MAK-2
Benzo[ghi]perylene 191-24-2																					EPA-D IARC-3
Benzo[c]phenanthrene 195-19-7																					IARC-2B

SUBSTANCE / CAS#	ACGIH® TLVs® TWA ppm	mg/m³	STEL/CEIL(C) ppm	mg/m³	OSHA PELs TWA ppm	mg/m³	STEL/CEIL(C) ppm	mg/m³	NIOSH RELs TWA ppm	mg/m³	STEL/CEIL(C) ppm	mg/m³	DFG MAKs TWA ppm	mg/m³	PEAK/CEIL(C) ppm	mg/m³	AIHA WEELs TWA ppm	mg/m³	STEL/CEIL(C) ppm	mg/m³	CARCINOGENICITY CATEGORY
Benzophenone 119-61-9																		0.5			IARC-2B
Benzo[a]pyrene 50-32-8	L; BEIp				0.2 *See* Coal tar pitch volatiles				0.1 Coal tar pitch volatiles, Cyclo-hexane-extractable fraction *See* Pocket Guide Apps. A and C				Skin; 2								EPA-B2 NTP-R IARC-1 TLV-A2 MAK-2 NIOSH-Ca
Benzo[e]pyrene 192-97-2																					IARC-3
Benzoquinone dioxime, p-isomer 105-11-3																					IARC-3
Benzotrichloride (Benzyl trichloride) 98-07-7	Skin		C 0.1	C 0.8									Skin								EPA-B2 TLV-A2 IARC-2A MAK-2 NTP-R
Benzoyl chloride 98-88-4			C 0.5	C 2.8													Skin; DSEN			C 5	IARC-2A MAK-3B TLV-A4
Benzoyl peroxide (Dibenzoyl peroxide) 94-36-0		5				5				5				5 I		I (1)					IARC-3 TLV-A4
Benzyl acetate 140-11-4	10	61																			IARC-3 TLV-A4
Benzyl alcohol 100-51-6																	10				

SUBSTANCE / CAS#	ACGIH® TLVs® TWA ppm	mg/m³	STEL/CEIL(C) ppm	mg/m³	OSHA PELs TWA ppm	mg/m³	STEL/CEIL(C) ppm	mg/m³	NIOSH RELs TWA ppm	mg/m³	STEL/CEIL(C) ppm	mg/m³	DFG MAKs TWA ppm	mg/m³	PEAK/CEIL(C) ppm	mg/m³	AIHA WEELs TWA ppm	mg/m³	STEL/CEIL(C) ppm	mg/m³	CARCINOGENICITY CATEGORY
Benzyl chloride 100-44-7	1	5.2			1	5					C 1* *15-min	C 5*		Skin							EPA-B2 IARC-2A MAK-2 TLV-A3
Benzylhemiformal 14548-60-8													releases Formaldehyde Sh								
Benzyl Violet 4B 1694-09-3																					IARC-2B
Beryllium [7440-41-7] **and compounds, as Be**		0.00005 I Skin; (SEN) NIC-DSEN; RSEN				0.002 *30 min peak per 8-hr shift	C 0.005; 0.025*			See Pocket Guide App. A	C 0.0005			Sah							EPA-B1; L*; NIOSH-Ca CBD** NTP-K IARC-1 TLV-A1 MAK-1 *inhaled **ingested
Biphenyl (Diphenyl) 92-52-4	0.2	1.3			0.2	1			0.2	1				Skin							EPA-D MAK-3B
Bismuth telluride, Undoped 1304-82-1		10				15*; 5** *Total dust **Respirable fraction				10*; 5** *Total dust **Respirable fraction											TLV-A4
Bismuth telluride, Se-doped, as Bi₂Te₃ 1304-82-1		5								5											TLV-A4
Bisphenol A (4,4'-Isopropylidenediphenol; BPA) 80-05-7													5 I SP; C		I (1)						
Bisphenol A diglycidyl-ether (4,4'-Isopropylidenediphenol diglycidyl ether) 1675-54-3														Skin; Sh							IARC-3 MAK-3A

SUBSTANCE CAS#	ACGIH® TLVs® TWA ppm	mg/m³	STEL/CEIL(C) ppm	mg/m³	OSHA PELs TWA ppm	mg/m³	STEL/CEIL(C) ppm	mg/m³	NIOSH RELs TWA ppm	mg/m³	STEL/CEIL(C) ppm	mg/m³	DFG MAKs TWA ppm	mg/m³	PEAK/CEIL(C) ppm	mg/m³	AIHA WEELs TWA ppm	mg/m³	STEL/CEIL(C) ppm	mg/m³	CARCINOGENICITY CATEGORY
Bisphenol A digly-cidyl methacrylate 1565-94-2														Sh							
Bisphenyl F diglycidal ether (o,o′-, o,p′-, p,p′-isomers) 54208-63-8; 57469-07-5; 2095-03-6														Sh							
Bisulfites																					IARC-3
Bithionol 97-18-7														SP							
Bleomycins 11056-06-7																					IARC-2B
Blue VRS 129-17-9																					IARC-3
Borate compounds, inorganic 1303-96-4; 1330-43-4; 10043-35-3; 12179-04-3	2 I		6 I						*See* Sodium tetraborate, anhydrous; Sodium tetraborate, decahydrate; and Sodium tetraborate, pentahydrate					10 I* 0.75 I** B*; C**	I (1)* I (1)**						TLV-A4
									*CAS: 10043-35-3 only **Tetraborates, as B												
Boron [7440-42-8] **and compounds**																					EPA-I

SUBSTANCE / CAS#	ACGIH® TLVs® TWA ppm	mg/m³	STEL/CEIL(C) ppm	mg/m³	OSHA PELs TWA ppm	mg/m³	STEL/CEIL(C) ppm	mg/m³	NIOSH RELs TWA ppm	mg/m³	STEL/CEIL(C) ppm	mg/m³	DFG MAKs TWA ppm	mg/m³	PEAK/CEIL(C) ppm	mg/m³	AIHA WEELs TWA ppm	mg/m³	STEL/CEIL(C) ppm	mg/m³	CARCINOGENICITY CATEGORY
Boron oxide 1303-86-2		10				15*				10											*Total dust
Boron tribromide 10294-33-4			C 1	C 10							C 1	C 10									
Boron trifluoride 7637-07-2			C 1	C 2.8			C 1	C 3			C 1	C 3									
Brilliant Blue FCF, disodium salt 3844-45-9																					IARC-3
Bromacil 314-40-9		10							1	10											TLV-A3
Bromate 15541-45-4																					EPA-L*; I**; B1 *oral route **inhalation
Bromelain 9001-00-7														Sa							
Brominated dibenzo-furans																					EPA-D
Bromine 7726-95-6	0.1	0.66	0.2	1.3	0.1	0.7			0.1	0.7	0.3	2									

SUBSTANCE CAS#	ACGIH® TLVs® TWA ppm	mg/m³	STEL/CEIL(C) ppm	mg/m³	OSHA PELs TWA ppm	mg/m³	STEL/CEIL(C) ppm	mg/m³	NIOSH RELs TWA ppm	mg/m³	STEL/CEIL(C) ppm	mg/m³	DFG MAKs TWA ppm	mg/m³	PEAK/CEIL(C) ppm	mg/m³	AIHA WEELs TWA ppm	mg/m³	STEL/CEIL(C) ppm	mg/m³	CARCINOGENICITY CATEGORY
Bromine pentafluoride 7789-30-2	0.1	0.72							0.1	0.7											
Bromobenzene 108-86-1																					EPA-II
Bromochloroacetic acid 5589-96-8																					IARC-2B
Bromochloroace-tonitrile 83463-62-1																					IARC-3
Bromodichloro-methane 75-27-4													Skin; 3B								EPA-B2 IARC-2B MAK-2 NTP-R
p-Bromodiphenyl ether 101-55-3																					EPA-D
Bromoform (Tribromomethane) 75-25-2	0.5	5.2			0.5	5			0.5	5											EPA-B2 IARC-3 MAK-3B TLV-A3
					Skin				Skin												
2,2-bis-(Bromomethyl)-1,3-propanediol, technical grade 3296-90-0																		0.2			IARC-2B NTP-R
2-Bromo-2-nitro-1,3-propanediol 52-51-7													Skin; Sh								

SUBSTANCE / CAS#	ACGIH® TLVs® TWA ppm	mg/m³	STEL/CEIL(C) ppm	mg/m³	OSHA PELs TWA ppm	mg/m³	STEL/CEIL(C) ppm	mg/m³	NIOSH RELs TWA ppm	mg/m³	STEL/CEIL(C) ppm	mg/m³	DFG MAKs TWA ppm	mg/m³	PEAK/CEIL(C) ppm	mg/m³	AIHA WEELs TWA ppm	mg/m³	STEL/CEIL(C) ppm	mg/m³	CARCINOGENICITY CATEGORY
1-Bromopropane 106-94-5	(10) NIC-0.1 NIC-A3	(50) NIC-0.5											Skin								MAK-2
Bromotrichloro-methane 75-62-7																					EPA-D
1,3-Butadiene 106-99-0	2	4.4			1 *See* 29 CFR 1910.1051; 29 CFR 1910.19(l)	2.21	5	11	*See* Pocket Guide App. A				2								EPA-CaH* NIOSH-Ca IARC-1 NTP-K MAK-1 TLV-A2 *inhaled
Butane, all isomers 106-97-8; 75-28-5			1000	2370					800 CAS: 106-97-8 only	1900			1000 D	2400	II (4)						
1,4-Butanediol diacrylate 1070-70-8													Sh								
1,4-Butanediol diglycidyl ether 2425-79-8													Sh								
1,4-Butanediol dimethacrylate 2082-81-7													Sh								
1,4-Butanediol dimethanesulfonate (Busulphan) 55-98-1																					IARC-1 NTP-K
1,4-Butane sultone 1633-83-6																					MAK-3B

SUBSTANCE / CAS#	ACGIH® TLVs® TWA ppm	mg/m³	STEL/CEIL(C) ppm	mg/m³	OSHA PELs TWA ppm	mg/m³	STEL/CEIL(C) ppm	mg/m³	NIOSH RELs TWA ppm	mg/m³	STEL/CEIL(C) ppm	mg/m³	DFG MAKs TWA ppm	mg/m³	PEAK/CEIL(C) ppm	mg/m³	AIHA WEELs TWA ppm	mg/m³	STEL/CEIL(C) ppm	mg/m³	CARCINOGENICITY CATEGORY
2,4-Butane sultone 1121-03-5																					MAK-2
n-Butanol (n-Butyl alcohol) 71-36-3	20	61			100	300					C 50	C 150	100	310	I (1)						EPA-D
						Skin								C							
sec-Butanol (sec-Butyl alcohol) 78-92-2	100	300			150	450			100	305	150	455									
tert-Butanol (tert-Butyl alcohol) 75-65-0	100	303			100	300			100	300	150	450	20	62	II (4)						TLV-A4
														C							
Butenes, all isomers 106-98-9; 107-01-7; 115-11-7; 590-18-1; 624-64-6; 25167-67-3	250	574																			TLV-A4* *CAS: 115-11-7 only
2-Butoxyethanol (EGBE) 111-76-2	20	97			50	240			5	24			10*	49	I (2)						EPA-NL IARC-3 MAK-4 TLV-A3
		BEI				Skin				Skin			*sum of the concentrations of EGBE and its acetate in air Skin; C								
2-Butoxyethyl acetate (EGBEA) 112-07-2	20	130							5	33			10*	66	I (2)						MAK-4 TLV-A3
													*sum of the concentrations of EGBE and its acetate in air Skin; C								
1-tert-Butoxy-2-propanol 57018-52-7																					IARC-3
														C							
n-Butyl acetate 123-86-4	150	713	200	950	150	710			150	710	200	950	100	480	I (2)						
														C							

SUBSTANCE / CAS#	ACGIH® TLVs® TWA ppm	mg/m³	STEL/CEIL(C) ppm	mg/m³	OSHA PELs TWA ppm	mg/m³	STEL/CEIL(C) ppm	mg/m³	NIOSH RELs TWA ppm	mg/m³	STEL/CEIL(C) ppm	mg/m³	DFG MAKs TWA ppm	mg/m³	PEAK/CEIL(C) ppm	mg/m³	AIHA WEELs TWA ppm	mg/m³	STEL/CEIL(C) ppm	mg/m³	CARCINOGENICITY CATEGORY
sec-Butyl acetate 105-46-4	200	950			200	950			200	950											
tert-Butyl acetate 540-88-5	200	950			200	950			200	950			20	96	II (4) C						
n-Butyl acrylate (Acrylic acid ester, n-Butyl ester) 141-32-2	2	11 (SEN) NIC-DSEN							10	55			2	11	I (2) Sh; C						IARC-3 TLV-A4
tert-Butyl acrylate 1663-39-4															Sh						
n-Butylamine 109-73-9			C 5 Skin	C 15			C 5 Skin	C 15			C 5 Skin	C 15	2	6.1	I (2) C 10 30 C						
sec-Butylamine 13952-84-6													2	6.1	I (2) C 10 30 C						
Butylated hydroxyanisole (BHA) 25013-16-5														20 I	II (1) C						IARC-2B MAK-3B NTP-R
Butylated hydroxytoluene (BHT; 2,6-Di-tert-butyl-p-cresol) 128-37-0		2 IFV								10				10 I	II (4) C						IARC-3 MAK-4 TLV-A4
4-tert-Butylbenzoic acid 98-73-7														2 I	II (2) Skin; D						

SUBSTANCE / CAS#	ACGIH® TLVs® TWA ppm	TWA mg/m³	STEL/CEIL(C) ppm	STEL/CEIL(C) mg/m³	OSHA PELs TWA ppm	TWA mg/m³	STEL/CEIL(C) ppm	STEL/CEIL(C) mg/m³	NIOSH RELs TWA ppm	TWA mg/m³	STEL/CEIL(C) ppm	STEL/CEIL(C) mg/m³	DFG MAKs TWA ppm	TWA mg/m³	PEAK/CEIL(C) ppm	PEAK/CEIL(C) mg/m³	AIHA WEELs TWA ppm	TWA mg/m³	STEL/CEIL(C) ppm	STEL/CEIL(C) mg/m³	CARCINOGENICITY CATEGORY
Butyl benzyl phthalate 85-68-7																					EPA-C IARC-3
Butyl carbitol acetate (Diethylene glycol monobutyl ether acetate) 124-17-4													10	85	I (1.5) C						
p-tert-Butylcatechol (4-[1,1-Dimethylethyl]-1,2-benzenediol) 98-29-3														Sh				Skin; DSEN	C 2		
tert-Butylchloride 507-20-0																					EPA-D
n-Butyl chloroformate (Chloroformic acid butyl ester) 592-34-7													0.2	1.1	I (2) C						
tert-Butyl chromate, as CrO₃ 1189-85-1			C 0.1	Skin	0.005	Skin See 29 CFR 1910.1026			0.001* *as Cr (VI) See Pocket Guide Apps. A and C												NIOSH-Ca
n-Butyl glycidyl ether (BGE) 2426-08-6	3	16 Skin; (SEN) NIC-DSEN			50	270				C 5.6* *15-min	C 30*			Skin; Sh; 2							MAK-3B
tert-Butyl glycidyl ether 7665-72-7														Skin; Sh							MAK-3B
n-Butyl lactate 138-22-7	5	30							5	25											

SUBSTANCE / CAS#	ACGIH® TLVs® TWA ppm	mg/m³	STEL/CEIL(C) ppm	mg/m³	OSHA PELs TWA ppm	mg/m³	STEL/CEIL(C) ppm	mg/m³	NIOSH RELs TWA ppm	mg/m³	STEL/CEIL(C) ppm	mg/m³	DFG MAKs TWA ppm	mg/m³	PEAK/CEIL(C) ppm	mg/m³	AIHA WEELs TWA ppm	mg/m³	STEL/CEIL(C) ppm	mg/m³	CARCINOGENICITY CATEGORY
n-Butyl mercaptan (Butanethiol) 109-79-5	0.5	1.8			10	35					C 0.5* *15-min	C 1.8*	0.5	1.9	II (2) C						
n-Butyl methacrylate 97-88-1														Sh							
o-sec-Butylphenol 89-72-5	5	31 Skin							5	30 Skin											
p-tert-Butylphenol 98-54-4													0.08	0.5 Skin; Sh; D	II (2)						
p-tert-Butyl phenyl glycidyl ether 3101-60-8														Sh							
p-tert-Butyltoluene 98-51-1	1	6.1			10	60			10	60	20	120									
iso-Butyl vinyl ether 109-53-5													20	83 D	I (1)						
Butynediol 110-65-6													0.1	0.36 Skin; Sh; C	I (1)						
Butyraldehyde 123-72-8																	25				

SUBSTANCE / CAS#	ACGIH® TLVs® TWA ppm	TWA mg/m³	STEL/CEIL(C) ppm	mg/m³	OSHA PELs TWA ppm	mg/m³	STEL/CEIL(C) ppm	mg/m³	NIOSH RELs TWA ppm	mg/m³	STEL/CEIL(C) ppm	mg/m³	DFG MAKs TWA ppm	mg/m³	PEAK/CEIL(C) ppm	mg/m³	AIHA WEELs TWA ppm	mg/m³	STEL/CEIL(C) ppm	mg/m³	CARCINOGENICITY CATEGORY
β-Butyrolactone 3068-88-0																					IARC-2B
γ-Butyrolactone 96-48-0														Skin							IARC-3
n-Butyronitrile 109-74-0									8	22											
Cacodylic acid 75-60-5																					EPA-D IARC-2B
Cadmium [7440-43-9] and compounds, as Cd	0.01	0.002 R BEI			0.005* *Table Z-2 for exclusions in 29 CFR 1910.1027 See 29 CFR 1910.1027				See Pocket Guide App. A												EPA-B1 OSHA-Ca IARC-1 TLV-A2 NIOSH-Ca NTP-K
Cadmium [7440-43-9] and inorganic compounds														Skin; 3A							MAK-1
Caffeic acid 331-39-5																					IARC-2B
Caffeine 58-08-2																					IARC-3
Calcium arsenate, as As 7778-44-1											C 0.002* *15-min See Pocket Guide App. A			See Arsenic and inorganic compounds							NIOSH-Ca

SUBSTANCE / CAS#	ACGIH® TLVs® TWA ppm	mg/m³	STEL/CEIL(C) ppm	mg/m³	OSHA PELs TWA ppm	mg/m³	STEL/CEIL(C) ppm	mg/m³	NIOSH RELs TWA ppm	mg/m³	STEL/CEIL(C) ppm	mg/m³	DFG MAKs TWA ppm	mg/m³	PEAK/CEIL(C) ppm	mg/m³	AIHA WEELs TWA ppm	mg/m³	STEL/CEIL(C) ppm	mg/m³	CARCINOGENICITY CATEGORY
Calcium carbonate (Limestone; Marble) 1317-65-3	TLV® withdrawn due to insufficient data				15*; 5** *Total dust **Respirable fraction				10*; 5** Includes CAS: 471-34-1 *Total dust **Respirable fraction												
Calcium chromate, as Cr 13756-19-0	0.001								See Chromic acid and chromates				See Chromium (VI) inorganic compounds, water-soluble								TLV-A2
Calcium cyanamide 156-62-7	0.5								0.5				1 I Skin; C		II (2)						TLV-A4
Calcium cyanide, as CN 592-01-8	See Hydrogen cyanide and Cyanide salts, as CN				See Cyanides				See Sodium cyanide				See Cyanides								
Calcium hydroxide 1305-62-0	5				15*; 5** *Total dust **Respirable fraction				5				1 I C		I (2)						
Calcium oxide 1305-78-8	2				5				2												
Calcium silicate 1344-95-2	10 synthetic nonfibrous E				15*; 5** *Total dust **Respirable fraction				10*; 5** *Total dust **Respirable fraction												TLV-A4
Calcium sodium meta-phosphate (fibrous dust) 23209-59-8																					MAK-3B
Calcium sulfate 7778-18-9; 10034-76-1; 10101-41-4; 13397-24-5	10 I				15*; 5** CAS: 7778-18-9 *Total dust **Respirable fraction				10*; 5** *Total dust **Respirable fraction				4 I 1.5 R C								

SUBSTANCE / CAS#	ACGIH® TLVs® TWA ppm	mg/m³	STEL/CEIL(C) ppm	mg/m³	OSHA PELs TWA ppm	mg/m³	STEL/CEIL(C) ppm	mg/m³	NIOSH RELs TWA ppm	mg/m³	STEL/CEIL(C) ppm	mg/m³	DFG MAKs TWA ppm	mg/m³	PEAK/CEIL(C) ppm	mg/m³	AIHA WEELs TWA ppm	mg/m³	STEL/CEIL(C) ppm	mg/m³	CARCINOGENICITY CATEGORY
Camphor, synthetic 76-22-2	2	12	3	19	2				2												TLV-A4
Cantharidin 56-25-7																					IARC-3
Caprolactam 105-60-2		5 IFV							0.22*	1**	0.66*	3**	5 I		I (2)						IARC-4 TLV-A5
									*vapor	**dust			C								
Captafol 2425-06-1		0.1								0.1											IARC-2A NIOSH-Ca NTP-R TLV-A4
	Skin								Skin See Pocket Guide App. A												
Captan 133-06-2		5 I								5											IARC-3 NIOSH-Ca TLV-A3
	(SEN) NIC-DSEN								See Pocket Guide App. A												
Carbaryl 63-25-2		0.5 IFV				5				5			5 I		II (4)						IARC-3 TLV-A4
	BEI_A; Skin												Skin								
Carbazole 86-74-8																					IARC-2B
Carbendazim 10605-21-7													10 I		II (4)						
												5; B									
3-Carbethoxypsoralen 20073-24-9																					IARC-3

SUBSTANCE / CAS#	ACGIH® TLVs® TWA ppm	mg/m³	STEL/CEIL(C) ppm	mg/m³	OSHA PELs TWA ppm	mg/m³	STEL/CEIL(C) ppm	mg/m³	NIOSH RELs TWA ppm	mg/m³	STEL/CEIL(C) ppm	mg/m³	DFG MAKs TWA ppm	mg/m³	PEAK/CEIL(C) ppm	mg/m³	AIHA WEELs TWA ppm	mg/m³	STEL/CEIL(C) ppm	mg/m³	CARCINOGENICITY CATEGORY
Carbofuran 1563-66-2	0.1 **IFV** BEI_A								0.1												TLV-A4
Carbon black 1333-86-4		3 **I**				3.5				3.5* *0.1 in presence of PAHs See Pocket Guide Apps. A and C				as Inhalable dust							IARC-2B TLV-A3 MAK-3B NIOSH-Ca* *in presence of PAHs
Carbon dioxide 124-38-9	5000	9000	30,000	54,000	5000	9000			5000	9000	30,000	54,000	5000	9100	II (2)						
Carbon disulfide 75-15-0	1	3.13 Skin; BEI			20 *30-min peak per 8-hr shift		C 30; 100*		1	3 Skin	10	30	5	16 Skin; B	II (2)						TLV-A4
Carbon monoxide 630-08-0	25	29 BEI			50	55			35	40	C 200	C 229	30	35 B	II (2)						
Carbon tetrabromide 558-13-4	0.1	1.4	0.3	4.1					0.1	1.4	0.3	4									
Carbon tetrachloride (Tetrachloromethane) 56-23-5	5	31 Skin	10	63	10 *5-min peak in any 3 hrs		C 25; 200*		See Pocket Guide App. A	2* *60-min	12.6*		0.5	3.2 Skin; C	II (2)						EPA-L NTP-R IARC-2B TLV-A2 MAK-4 NIOSH-Ca
Carbonyl fluoride 353-50-4	2	5.4	5	13					2	5	5	15									
Carbonyl sulfide 463-58-1	5	12																			

SUBSTANCE / CAS#	ACGIH® TLVs® TWA ppm	mg/m³	STEL/CEIL(C) ppm	mg/m³	OSHA PELs TWA ppm	mg/m³	STEL/CEIL(C) ppm	mg/m³	NIOSH RELs TWA ppm	mg/m³	STEL/CEIL(C) ppm	mg/m³	DFG MAKs TWA ppm	mg/m³	PEAK/CEIL(C) ppm	mg/m³	AIHA WEELs TWA ppm	mg/m³	STEL/CEIL(C) ppm	mg/m³	CARCINOGENICITY CATEGORY
N-Carboxyanthranilic anhydride 118-48-9														Sh							
Carmoisine 3567-69-9																					IARC-3
Carrageenan, degraded 53973-98-1																					IARC-2B
Carrageenan, native 9000-07-1																					IARC-3
Catechol (Pyrocatechol) 120-80-9	5	23		Skin					5	20		Skin									IARC-2B TLV-A3
Cellulases														Sa							
Cellulose 9004-34-6		10			15*; 5**			*Total dust **Respirable fraction	10*; 5**			*Total dust **Respirable fraction									
Cereal flour dusts (Rye, wheat)														Sa							
Cerium oxide and cerium compounds 1306-38-3																					EPA-I

SUBSTANCE / CAS#	ACGIH® TLVs® TWA ppm	TWA mg/m³	STEL/CEIL(C) ppm	mg/m³	OSHA PELs TWA ppm	TWA mg/m³	STEL/CEIL(C) ppm	mg/m³	NIOSH RELs TWA ppm	TWA mg/m³	STEL/CEIL(C) ppm	mg/m³	DFG MAKs TWA ppm	TWA mg/m³	PEAK/CEIL(C) ppm	mg/m³	AIHA WEELs TWA ppm	TWA mg/m³	STEL/CEIL(C) ppm	mg/m³	CARCINOGENICITY CATEGORY
Cesium hydroxide 21351-79-1	2								2												
Cetylmercaptan (1-Hexadecanethiol) 2917-26-2											C 0.5* *15-min	C 5.3*									
Chimney sweeping																					IARC-1
Chloral 75-87-6																					IARC-2A
Chloral hydrate 302-17-0																					EPA-C; CBD* IARC-2A *oral
Chlorambucil 305-03-3																					IARC-1 NTP-K
Chloramine 10599-90-3																					EPA-D IARC-3
Chloramphenicol 56-75-7																		0.5			IARC-2A NTP-R
Chlordane 57-74-9	0.5 Skin				0.5 Skin				0.5 Skin *See* Pocket Guide App. A				0.5 I Skin		II (8)						EPA-L*; B2 NIOSH-Ca IARC-2B TLV-A3 MAK-3B *CAS: 12789-03-6

SUBSTANCE CAS#	ACGIH® TLVs® TWA ppm	ACGIH® TLVs® TWA mg/m³	ACGIH® TLVs® STEL/CEIL(C) ppm	ACGIH® TLVs® STEL/CEIL(C) mg/m³	OSHA PELs TWA ppm	OSHA PELs TWA mg/m³	OSHA PELs STEL/CEIL(C) ppm	OSHA PELs STEL/CEIL(C) mg/m³	NIOSH RELs TWA ppm	NIOSH RELs TWA mg/m³	NIOSH RELs STEL/CEIL(C) ppm	NIOSH RELs STEL/CEIL(C) mg/m³	DFG MAKs TWA ppm	DFG MAKs TWA mg/m³	DFG MAKs PEAK/CEIL(C) ppm	DFG MAKs PEAK/CEIL(C) mg/m³	AIHA WEELs TWA ppm	AIHA WEELs TWA mg/m³	AIHA WEELs STEL/CEIL(C) ppm	AIHA WEELs STEL/CEIL(C) mg/m³	CARCINOGENICITY CATEGORY
Chlordecone 143-50-0										0.001 *See* Pocket Guide App. A				Skin							EPA-L* NIOSH-Ca IARC-2B NTP-R MAK-2 *oral
Chlordimeform 6164-98-3																					IARC-3
Chlorendic acid 115-28-6																					IARC-2B NTP-R
Chlorinated biphenyls: higher chlorinated (≥ 4 Cl) biphenyls														0.003 **I*** *(PCB 28 + PCB 52 + PCB 101 + PCB 138 + PCB 153 + PCB 180) − 5 Skin; B5	II (8)						MAK-4
Chlorinated biphenyls: mono-, di-, trichlorinated biphenyls														Skin; 3A							MAK-3B
Chlorinated camphene (Toxaphene) 8001-35-2	0.5		1	Skin	0.5			Skin		Skin *See* Pocket Guide App. A				Skin							EPA-B2 NTP-R IARC-2B TLV-A3 MAK-2 NIOSH-Ca
o-Chlorinated diphenyl oxide 31242-93-0	0.5				0.5				0.5					several CAS Nos., e.g., 55720-99-5 Skin							
Chlorinated drinking water																					IARC-3
Chlorinated naphthalenes														Skin							

SUBSTANCE CAS#	ACGIH® TLVs® TWA ppm	mg/m³	STEL/CEIL(C) ppm	mg/m³	OSHA PELs TWA ppm	mg/m³	STEL/CEIL(C) ppm	mg/m³	NIOSH RELs TWA ppm	mg/m³	STEL/CEIL(C) ppm	mg/m³	DFG MAKs TWA ppm	mg/m³	PEAK/CEIL(C) ppm	mg/m³	AIHA WEELs TWA ppm	mg/m³	STEL/CEIL(C) ppm	mg/m³	CARCINOGENICITY CATEGORY
Chlorinated paraffins, 20%–70% chlorine																					IARC-2B* MAK-3B NTP-R* *60%
α-Chlorinated toluenes, mixture of benzoyl chloride, benzyl chloride, benzyl dichloride and benzyl trichloride													Skin								IARC-2A MAK-1
Chlorine 7782-50-5	0.5	1.5	1	2.9			C 1	C 3			C 0.5* *15-min	C 1.45*	0.5	1.5	I (1) C						TLV-A4
Chlorine dioxide 10049-04-4	0.1	0.28	0.3	0.83	0.1	0.3			0.1	0.3	0.3	0.9	0.1	0.28	I (1) D						EPA-CBD; D
Chlorine trifluoride 7790-91-2			C 0.1	C 0.38			C 0.1	C 0.4			C 0.1	C 0.4									
Chlorite, sodium salt 7758-19-2																					EPA-CBD; D IARC-3
Chloroacetaldehyde 107-20-0			C 1	C 3.2			C 1	C 3			C 1	C 3	Skin								MAK-3B
2-Chloroacetamide 79-07-2													Skin; Sh								

SUBSTANCE / CAS#	ACGIH® TLVs® TWA ppm	mg/m³	STEL/CEIL(C) ppm	mg/m³	OSHA PELs TWA ppm	mg/m³	STEL/CEIL(C) ppm	mg/m³	NIOSH RELs TWA ppm	mg/m³	STEL/CEIL(C) ppm	mg/m³	DFG MAKs TWA ppm	mg/m³	PEAK/CEIL(C) ppm	mg/m³	AIHA WEELs TWA ppm	mg/m³	STEL/CEIL(C) ppm	mg/m³	CARCINOGENICITY CATEGORY
Chloroacetamide-N-methylol (CAM) 2832-19-1														Sh							MAK-3B
Chloroacetic acid, methyl ester (Methyl chloroacetate) 96-34-4													1	4.5	I (1)			Skin; Sh; C			
Chloroacetone 78-95-5			C 1	C 3.8																	
		Skin																			
Chloroacetonitrile 107-14-2																					IARC-3
2-Chloroacetophenone (Phenacyl chloride) 532-27-4	0.05	0.32			0.05	0.3			0.05	0.3											TLV-A4
Chloroacetyl chloride 79-04-9	0.05	0.23	0.15	0.69					0.05	0.2				Skin							
		Skin																			
2-Chloroacrylonitrile 920-37-6																					MAK-3B
Chloroaniline, m-isomer 108-42-9														Skin; Sh							
Chloroaniline, o-isomer 95-51-2														Skin							

OCCUPATIONAL EXPOSURE VALUES

SUBSTANCE / CAS#	ACGIH® TLVs® TWA ppm	mg/m³	STEL/CEIL(C) ppm	mg/m³	OSHA PELs TWA ppm	mg/m³	STEL/CEIL(C) ppm	mg/m³	NIOSH RELs TWA ppm	mg/m³	STEL/CEIL(C) ppm	mg/m³	DFG MAKs TWA ppm	mg/m³	PEAK/CEIL(C) ppm	mg/m³	AIHA WEELs TWA ppm	mg/m³	STEL/CEIL(C) ppm	mg/m³	CARCINOGENICITY CATEGORY
Chloroaniline, p-isomer 106-47-8													Skin; Sh								IARC-2B MAK-2
Chlorobenzene (Monochlorobenzene) 108-90-7	10	46	BEI		75	350							10	47	II (2) C						EPA-D TLV-A3
Chlorobenzilate 510-15-6																					IARC-3
Chlorobenzotrichloride, p-isomer 5216-25-1													Skin								MAK-2
Chlorobenzylidene malononitrile, o-isomer 2698-41-1			C 0.05 Skin	C 0.39	0.05	0.4					C 0.05 Skin	C 0.4									TLV-A4
Chlorobromomethane (Bromochloromethane) 74-97-5	200	1060			200	1050			200	1050			Skin								EPA-D MAK-3B
1-Chlorobutane 109-69-3																					EPA-D
2-Chlorobutane 78-86-4																					EPA-D
p-Chloro-m-cresol 59-50-7													Sh								

SUBSTANCE / CAS#	ACGIH® TLVs® TWA ppm	mg/m³	STEL/CEIL(C) ppm	mg/m³	OSHA PELs TWA ppm	mg/m³	STEL/CEIL(C) ppm	mg/m³	NIOSH RELs TWA ppm	mg/m³	STEL/CEIL(C) ppm	mg/m³	DFG MAKs TWA ppm	mg/m³	PEAK/CEIL(C) ppm	mg/m³	AIHA WEELs TWA ppm	mg/m³	STEL/CEIL(C) ppm	mg/m³	CARCINOGENICITY CATEGORY
Chlorocyclopentadiene 41851-50-7																					EPA-D
Chlorodibromo-methane 124-48-1																					EPA-C IARC-3
3-Chloro-4-(dichloro-methyl)-5-hydroxy-2 (5H)-furanone 77439-76-0																					IARC-2B
1-Chloro-1,1-difluoro-ethane (FC-142b) 75-68-3													1000	4200	II (8) D		1000				
Chlorodifluoromethane (FC-22) 75-45-6	1000	3540							1000	3500	1250	4375	500	1800	II (8) C						IARC-3 TLV-A4
1-Chloro-2,4-dinitrobenzene 97-00-7															Sh						
Chlorodiphenyl, 42% chlorine 53469-21-9	1 Skin				1 Skin				0.001 See Pocket Guide App. A				See Chlorinated biphenyls								NIOSH-Ca
Chlorodiphenyl, 54% chlorine 11097-69-1	0.5 Skin				0.5 Skin				0.001 See Pocket Guide App. A				See Chlorinated biphenyls								NIOSH-Ca TLV-A3
bis(2-Chloroethoxy)-methane 111-91-1																					EPA-D

SUBSTANCE CAS#	ACGIH® TLVs®				OSHA PELs				NIOSH RELs				DFG MAKs				AIHA WEELs				CARCINOGENICITY CATEGORY
	TWA		STEL/CEIL(C)		TWA		STEL/CEIL(C)		TWA		STEL/CEIL(C)		TWA		PEAK/CEIL(C)		TWA		STEL/CEIL(C)		
	ppm	mg/m³	ppm	mg/m³	ppm	mg/m³	ppm	mg/m³	ppm	mg/m³	ppm	mg/m³	ppm	mg/m³	ppm	mg/m³	ppm	mg/m³	ppm	mg/m³	
1-(2-Chloroethyl)-3-cyclohexyl-1-nitrosourea (CCNU) 13010-47-4																					IARC-1 NTP-R
1-(2-Chloroethyl)-3-(4-methylcyclohexyl)-1-nitrosourea (Methyl-CCNU; Semustine) 13909-09-6																					IARC-1 NTP-K
N,N-bis(2-Chloroethyl)-2-naphthylamine (Chlornaphazine) 494-03-1																					IARC-1
bis(Chloroethyl)nitrosourea (BCNU) 154-93-8																					IARC-2A NTP-R
tris(2-Chloroethyl) phosphate 115-96-8																					IARC-3
Chlorofluoromethane (FC-31) 593-70-4																					IARC-3 MAK-2
Chloroform (Trichloromethane) 67-66-3	10	49					C 50	C 240			2* *60-min See Pocket Guide App. A	9.78*	0.5	2.5	II (2) Skin; C						EPA-B2; NIOSH-Ca L; NL NTP-R IARC-2B TLV-A3 MAK-4
Chloroformic acid butyl ester 543-27-1; 592-34-7													0.2	1.1	I (2) C						

SUBSTANCE / CAS#	ACGIH® TLVs®				OSHA PELs				NIOSH RELs				DFG MAKs				AIHA WEELs				CARCINOGENICITY CATEGORY
	TWA		STEL/CEIL(C)		TWA		STEL/CEIL(C)		TWA		STEL/CEIL(C)		TWA		PEAK/CEIL(C)		TWA		STEL/CEIL(C)		
	ppm	mg/m³	ppm	mg/m³	ppm	mg/m³	ppm	mg/m³	ppm	mg/m³	ppm	mg/m³	ppm	mg/m³	ppm	mg/m³	ppm	mg/m³	ppm	mg/m³	
N-Chloroformyl-morpholine 15159-40-7																					MAK-2
bis-(2-Chloroiso-propyl)ether 39638-32-9																	3				
1,2-bis(Chlorometh-oxy)ethane 13483-18-6																					IARC-3
1,4-bis(Chlorometh-oxymethyl)benzene 56894-91-8																					IARC-3
1,2,3-tris(Chlorometh-oxy)propane 38571-73-2																					IARC-3
5-Chloro-2-methyl-2,3-dihydroisothiazol-3-one [26172-55-4] and 2-Methyl-2,3-dihydroiso-thiazol-3-one [2682-20-4] mixture in ratio 3:1 Sh; C													0.2 I		I (2)						
bis(2-Chloro-1-methyl-ethyl)ether 108-60-1																					IARC-3
bis(Chloromethyl)ether 542-88-1	0.001	0.0047			*See* 29 CFR 1910.1003				*See* Pocket Guide App. A												EPA-A NTP-K* IARC-1* OSHA-Ca MAK-1 TLV-A1 NIOSH-Ca *includes technical grades

SUBSTANCE / CAS#	ACGIH® TLVs® TWA ppm	ACGIH® TLVs® TWA mg/m³	ACGIH® TLVs® STEL/CEIL(C) ppm	ACGIH® TLVs® STEL/CEIL(C) mg/m³	OSHA PELs TWA ppm	OSHA PELs TWA mg/m³	OSHA PELs STEL/CEIL(C) ppm	OSHA PELs STEL/CEIL(C) mg/m³	NIOSH RELs TWA ppm	NIOSH RELs TWA mg/m³	NIOSH RELs STEL/CEIL(C) ppm	NIOSH RELs STEL/CEIL(C) mg/m³	DFG MAKs TWA ppm	DFG MAKs TWA mg/m³	DFG MAKs PEAK/CEIL(C) ppm	DFG MAKs PEAK/CEIL(C) mg/m³	AIHA WEELs TWA ppm	AIHA WEELs TWA mg/m³	AIHA WEELs STEL/CEIL(C) ppm	AIHA WEELs STEL/CEIL(C) mg/m³	CARCINOGENICITY CATEGORY
Chloromethyl methyl ether (CMME; Methyl chloro-methyl ether) 107-30-2		L			*See* 29 CFR 1910.1003				*See* Pocket Guide App. A												EPA-A NTP-K* IARC-1* OSHA-Ca MAK-1 TLV-A2 NIOSH-Ca *includes technical grades
1-Chloro-2-methylpro-pene (Dimethylvinyl chloride) 513-37-1																					IARC-2B NTP-R
3-Chloro-2-methyl-propene 563-47-3																					IARC-3 MAK-3B NTP-R
1-Chloro-1-nitropropane 600-25-9	2	10			20	100			2	10											
Chloropentafluoro-ethane 76-15-3	1000	6320							1000	6320											
4-Chloro-m-phenyl-enediamine 5131-60-2																					IARC-3
4-Chloro-o-phenyl-enediamine 95-83-0																					IARC-2B NTP-R
4-Chlorophenyl isocyanate 104-12-1																					MAK-3B
p-Chlorophenyl methyl sulfide 123-09-1																					EPA-D

SUBSTANCE / CAS#	ACGIH® TLVs® TWA ppm	TWA mg/m³	STEL/CEIL(C) ppm	mg/m³	OSHA PELs TWA ppm	mg/m³	STEL/CEIL(C) ppm	mg/m³	NIOSH RELs TWA ppm	mg/m³	STEL/CEIL(C) ppm	mg/m³	DFG MAKs TWA ppm	mg/m³	PEAK/CEIL(C) ppm	mg/m³	AIHA WEELs TWA ppm	mg/m³	STEL/CEIL(C) ppm	mg/m³	CARCINOGENICITY CATEGORY
p-Chlorophenyl methyl sulfone 98-57-7																					EPA-D
p-Chlorophenyl methyl sulfoxide 934-73-6																					EPA-D
Chloropicrin (Trichloronitromethane) 76-06-2	0.1	0.67			0.1	0.7			0.1	0.7			0.1	0.68	I (1)						TLV-A4
2-Chloropropane 75-29-6																	50				
1-Chloro-2-propanol [127-00-4] and 2-Chloro-1-propanol [78-89-7]	1	4																			TLV-A4
		Skin																			
β-Chloroprene (2-Chloro-1,3-butadiene) 126-99-8	10	36			25	90					C 1*	C 3.6*									EPA-L NIOSH-Ca IARC-2B NTP-R MAK-2
		Skin				Skin			*15-min See Pocket Guide App. A					Skin							
Chloropropham 101-21-3																					IARC-3
2-Chloropropionic acid 598-78-7	0.1	0.44																			
		Skin																			
Chloroquine 54-05-7																					IARC-3

SUBSTANCE / CAS#	ACGIH® TLVs® TWA ppm	mg/m³	STEL/CEIL(C) ppm	mg/m³	OSHA PELs TWA ppm	mg/m³	STEL/CEIL(C) ppm	mg/m³	NIOSH RELs TWA ppm	mg/m³	STEL/CEIL(C) ppm	mg/m³	DFG MAKs TWA ppm	mg/m³	PEAK/CEIL(C) ppm	mg/m³	AIHA WEELs TWA ppm	mg/m³	STEL/CEIL(C) ppm	mg/m³	CARCINOGENICITY CATEGORY
Chlorostyrene, o-isomer 2039-87-4	50	283	75	425					50	285	75	428									
Chlorosulfonic acid 7790-94-5																				C 0.1	
2-Chloro-1,1,1,2-tetrafluoroethane 2837-89-0																	1000				
Chlorothalonil 1897-45-6															Sh						IARC-2B MAK-3B
Chlorotoluene, o-isomer 95-49-8	50	259							50	250	75	375									
4-Chloro-o-toluidine 95-69-2															Skin; 3A						IARC-2A MAK-1 NTP-R
5-Chloro-o-toluidine 95-79-4																					IARC-3 MAK-3B
p-Chloro-o-toluidine hydrochloride 3165-93-3																					NTP-R
2-Chloro-1,1,1-trifluoroethane 75-88-7																					IARC-3

SUBSTANCE / CAS#	ACGIH® TLVs® TWA ppm	mg/m³	STEL/CEIL(C) ppm	mg/m³	OSHA PELs TWA ppm	mg/m³	STEL/CEIL(C) ppm	mg/m³	NIOSH RELs TWA ppm	mg/m³	STEL/CEIL(C) ppm	mg/m³	DFG MAKs TWA ppm	mg/m³	PEAK/CEIL(C)	AIHA WEELs TWA ppm	mg/m³	STEL/CEIL(C) ppm	mg/m³	CARCINOGENICITY CATEGORY
Chlorotrifluoro-ethylene 79-38-9																5				
Chlorotrifluoromethane (FC-13) 75-72-9													1000	4300	II (8) D					
Chlorozotocin 54749-90-5																				IARC-2A NTP-R
Chlorpromazine 50-53-3															SP					
Chlorpyrifos 2921-88-2	0.1 IFV								0.2	0.6										TLV-A4
	Skin; BEI$_A$								Skin											
Cholesterol 57-88-5																				IARC-3
Chromic acid [7738-94-5] and chromates	See Chromium (VI) inorganic compounds, water-soluble						C 0.1* *as CrO₃		0.001* *as Cr See Pocket Guide Apps. A and C				See Chromium (VI) inorganic compounds, water-soluble							NIOSH-Ca
Chromite ore processing (Chromate), as Cr	0.05																			TLV-A1
Chromium (II) inorganic compounds, as Cr						0.5				0.5 See Pocket Guide App. C										

47

SUBSTANCE / CAS#	ACGIH® TLVs® TWA ppm	ACGIH® TLVs® TWA mg/m³	ACGIH® TLVs® STEL/CEIL(C) ppm	ACGIH® TLVs® STEL/CEIL(C) mg/m³	OSHA PELs TWA ppm	OSHA PELs TWA mg/m³	OSHA PELs STEL/CEIL(C) ppm	OSHA PELs STEL/CEIL(C) mg/m³	NIOSH RELs TWA ppm	NIOSH RELs TWA mg/m³	NIOSH RELs STEL/CEIL(C) ppm	NIOSH RELs STEL/CEIL(C) mg/m³	DFG MAKs TWA ppm	DFG MAKs TWA mg/m³	DFG MAKs PEAK/CEIL(C) ppm	DFG MAKs PEAK/CEIL(C) mg/m³	AIHA WEELs TWA ppm	AIHA WEELs TWA mg/m³	AIHA WEELs STEL/CEIL(C) ppm	AIHA WEELs STEL/CEIL(C) mg/m³	CARCINOGENICITY CATEGORY
Chromium (III) 16065-83-1																					EPA-D*, CBD* IARC-3** *insoluble salts **compounds
Chromium (III) inorganic compounds, as Cr 7440-47-3		0.5				0.5				0.5 See Pocket Guide App. C				Sh* *does not apply to Cr (III) oxide and similar poorly soluble Cr (III) compounds							EPA-D; CBD TLV-A4
Chromium (VI) 18540-29-9						0.005* *compounds, as Cr (VI) See 29 CFR 1910.1026															EPA-A*; K*; D**; CBD** IARC-1 *inhalation **oral
Chromium (VI) inorganic compounds, water-soluble		0.05* *as Cr BEI				0.005* *as Cr (VI) See 29 CFR 1910.1026			0.001* *as Cr See Pocket Guide Apps. A and C					Inhalable fraction Skin*; Sh**; 2 *the chromates of Ba, Pb, Sr, and Zn are not designated with Skin **BaCrO₄ and PbCrO₄ are not designated with Sh							EPA-A*; K*; NIOSH-Ca D**; CBD** IARC-1 TLV-A1 MAK-1 *inhalation **oral
Chromium (VI) inorganic compounds, insoluble		0.01* *as Cr				0.005* *as Cr (VI) See 29 CFR 1910.1026			0.001* *as Cr See Pocket Guide Apps. A and C					Inhalable fraction Skin*; Sh**; 2 *the chromates of Ba, Pb, Sr, and Zn are not designated with Skin **BaCrO₄ and PbCrO₄ are not designated with Sh							EPA-A*; K*; NIOSH-Ca D**; CBD** NTP-K IARC-1 TLV-A1 MAK-1 *inhalation **oral
Chromium metal 7440-47-3		0.5				1				0.5 See Pocket Guide App. C											EPA-A*; K*; IARC-3 D**; CBD** TLV-A4 *inhalation **oral
Chromyl chloride 14977-61-8	0.025	0.16							See Chromium (VI) inorganic compounds, water-soluble				See Chromium (VI) inorganic compounds, water-soluble								IARC-2 MAK-1 NIOSH-Ca NTP-K

Note: The DFG MAKs "Inhalable fraction / Skin*; Sh**; 2" and related footnotes appear under the DFG MAKs column group. The "See Chromium (VI) inorganic compounds, water-soluble" note for Chromyl chloride appears under NIOSH RELs and DFG MAKs columns.

SUBSTANCE / CAS#	ACGIH® TLVs® TWA ppm	mg/m³	STEL/CEIL(C) ppm	mg/m³	OSHA PELs TWA ppm	mg/m³	STEL/CEIL(C) ppm	mg/m³	NIOSH RELs TWA ppm	mg/m³	STEL/CEIL(C) ppm	mg/m³	DFG MAKs TWA ppm	mg/m³	PEAK/CEIL(C)	AIHA WEELs TWA ppm	mg/m³	STEL/CEIL(C) ppm	mg/m³	CARCINOGENICITY CATEGORY
Chrysene 218-01-9	L; BEI_P				0.2 *See* Coal tar pitch volatiles				0.1* *Cyclohexane-extractable fraction* *See* Pocket Guide Apps. A and C						Skin					EPA-B2 NIOSH-Ca IARC-2B TLV-A3 MAK-2
Chrysoidine 532-82-1																				IARC-3
CI Acid Orange 3 6373-74-6																				IARC-3
CI Acid Red 114 6459-94-5																				IARC-2B
CI Basic Red 9 569-61-9																				IARC-2B NTP-R
CI Direct Blue 15 2429-74-5																				IARC-2B
Cimetidine 51481-61-9																				IARC-3
Cinnamaldehyde 104-55-2															Sh					
Cinnamyl alcohol 104-54-1															Sh					

SUBSTANCE / CAS#	ACGIH® TLVs® TWA ppm	ACGIH® TLVs® TWA mg/m³	ACGIH® TLVs® STEL/CEIL(C) ppm	ACGIH® TLVs® STEL/CEIL(C) mg/m³	OSHA PELs TWA ppm	OSHA PELs TWA mg/m³	OSHA PELs STEL/CEIL(C) ppm	OSHA PELs STEL/CEIL(C) mg/m³	NIOSH RELs TWA ppm	NIOSH RELs TWA mg/m³	NIOSH RELs STEL/CEIL(C) ppm	NIOSH RELs STEL/CEIL(C) mg/m³	DFG MAKs TWA ppm	DFG MAKs TWA mg/m³	DFG MAKs PEAK/CEIL(C) ppm	DFG MAKs PEAK/CEIL(C) mg/m³	AIHA WEELs TWA ppm	AIHA WEELs TWA mg/m³	AIHA WEELs STEL/CEIL(C) ppm	AIHA WEELs STEL/CEIL(C) mg/m³	CARCINOGENICITY CATEGORY
Cinnamyl anthranilate / 87-29-6																					IARC-3
CI Pigment Red 3 / 2425-85-6																					IARC-3
Cisplatin / 15663-27-1																					IARC-2A NTP-R
Citral / 5392-40-5	5 **IFV** Skin; (SEN) NIC-DSEN																				TLV-A4
Citrinin / 518-75-2																					IARC-3
Citrus Red No. 2 / 6358-53-8																					IARC-2B
Clofibrate / 637-07-0																					IARC-3
Clomiphene citrate / 50-41-9																					IARC-3
Clopidol / 2971-90-6	3 **IFV**					15*; 5** *Total dust **Respirable fraction				10*; 5** *Total dust **Respirable fraction		20*								TLV-A4

SUBSTANCE / CAS#	ACGIH® TLVs® TWA ppm	TWA mg/m³	STEL/CEIL(C) ppm	mg/m³	OSHA PELs TWA ppm	TWA mg/m³	STEL/CEIL(C) ppm	mg/m³	NIOSH RELs TWA ppm	TWA mg/m³	STEL/CEIL(C) ppm	mg/m³	DFG MAKs TWA ppm	TWA mg/m³	PEAK/CEIL(C) ppm	mg/m³	AIHA WEELs TWA ppm	TWA mg/m³	STEL/CEIL(C) ppm	mg/m³	CARCINOGENICITY CATEGORY
Coal dust, anthracite; bituminous or lignite		0.4 R* 0.9 R** *Anthracite **Bituminous or lignite				2.4* $\dfrac{10 \text{ mg/m}^3 {}^{**}}{\% \text{ SiO}_2 + 2}$ *< 5% SiO₂, resp. Quartz fraction ** ≥ 5% SiO₂, resp. Quartz fraction				1* 0.9** *measured according to MSHA method (CPSU) **measured according to ISO/CEN/ACGIH® criteria See Pocket Guide App. C										IARC-3 MAK-3B* TLV-A4 *coal mine dust
Coal gasification																					IARC-1
Coal-tar distillation																					IARC-1
Coal-tar pitch																					IARC-1 NTP-K
Coal tar pitch volatiles, as benzene soluble aerosol 65996-93-2	0.2	BEI_P			0.2				0.1* *Cyclohexane-extractable fraction See Pocket Guide Apps. A and C												IARC-1 NIOSH-Ca NTP-K TLV-A1
Cobalt, alloys													Cobalt alloys containing bio-available cobalt, see Cobalt and compounds								
Cobalt [7440-48-4] and compounds													as Inhalable fraction Skin; Sah; 3A								IARC-2B MAK-2
Cobalt [7440-48-4] and inorganic compounds, as Co	0.02	BEI			0.1* *for metal dust and fume				0.05* *for metal dust and fume												TLV-A3

SUBSTANCE / CAS#	ACGIH® TLVs® TWA ppm	ACGIH® TLVs® TWA mg/m³	ACGIH® TLVs® STEL/CEIL(C) ppm	ACGIH® TLVs® STEL/CEIL(C) mg/m³	OSHA PELs TWA ppm	OSHA PELs TWA mg/m³	OSHA PELs STEL/CEIL(C) ppm	OSHA PELs STEL/CEIL(C) mg/m³	NIOSH RELs TWA ppm	NIOSH RELs TWA mg/m³	NIOSH RELs STEL/CEIL(C) ppm	NIOSH RELs STEL/CEIL(C) mg/m³	DFG MAKs TWA ppm	DFG MAKs TWA mg/m³	DFG MAKs PEAK/CEIL(C) ppm	DFG MAKs PEAK/CEIL(C) mg/m³	AIHA WEELs TWA ppm	AIHA WEELs TWA mg/m³	AIHA WEELs STEL/CEIL(C) ppm	AIHA WEELs STEL/CEIL(C) mg/m³	CARCINOGENICITY CATEGORY
Cobalt [7440-48-4] with tungsten carbide [12070-12-1]																					IARC-2A NTP-R* *powders and hard metals
Cobalt carbonyl, as Co 10210-68-1		0.1								0.1											IARC-2B
Cobalt hydrocarbonyl, as Co 16842-03-8		0.1								0.1											IARC-2B
Cobalt sulfate 10124-43-3														See Cobalt and compounds							IARC-2B* NTP-R *and other soluble Cobalt (II) salts
Coke oven emissions						0.15* *Benzene-soluble fraction See 29 CFR 1910.1029				0.2* *Benzene-soluble fraction See Pocket Guide Apps. A and C										EPA-A MAK-1 NIOSH-Ca NTP-K OSHA-Ca
Coke production																					IARC-1
Copper, dusts and mists, as Cu 7440-50-8		1				1				1											EPA-D
Copper, fume, as Cu 7440-50-8		0.2				0.1				0.1											EPA-D
Copper [7440-50-8] and its inorganic compounds														0.1 I	II (2) C						EPA-D

SUBSTANCE / CAS#	ACGIH® TLVs® TWA ppm	mg/m³	STEL/CEIL(C) ppm	mg/m³	OSHA PELs TWA ppm	mg/m³	STEL/CEIL(C) ppm	mg/m³	NIOSH RELs TWA ppm	mg/m³	STEL/CEIL(C) ppm	mg/m³	DFG MAKs TWA ppm	mg/m³	PEAK/CEIL(C) ppm	mg/m³	AIHA WEELs TWA ppm	mg/m³	STEL/CEIL(C) ppm	mg/m³	CARCINOGENICITY CATEGORY
Copper-8-hydroxy-quinoline 10380-28-6																					IARC-3
Coronene 191-07-1																					IARC-3
Cotton dust, in textile mill waste house operations, in yarn manufacturing, or from "lower-grade washed cotton"						0.5* *Lint-free respirable dust, as measured by vert. elutriator. See 29 CFR 1910.1043														
Cotton dust, in textile slashing and weaving operations						0.75* *Lint-free respirable dust, as measured by vert. elutriator. See 29 CFR 1910.1043														
Cotton dust, in yarn manufacturing and cotton washing operations						0.2* *Lint-free respirable dust, as measured by vert. elutriator. See 29 CFR 1910.1043														
Cotton dust, raw, untreated		0.1 T				1* *Resp. dust, measured by vert. elutriator (cotton waste processing oper.)				< 0.2 See Pocket Guide App. C				1.5 I C	I (1)						TLV-A4
Coumaphos 56-72-4		0.05 IFV Skin; BEI_A																			TLV-A4
Coumarin 91-64-5																					IARC-3

SUBSTANCE / CAS#	ACGIH® TLVs® TWA ppm	ACGIH® TLVs® TWA mg/m³	ACGIH® TLVs® STEL/CEIL(C) ppm	ACGIH® TLVs® STEL/CEIL(C) mg/m³	OSHA PELs TWA ppm	OSHA PELs TWA mg/m³	OSHA PELs STEL/CEIL(C) ppm	OSHA PELs STEL/CEIL(C) mg/m³	NIOSH RELs TWA ppm	NIOSH RELs TWA mg/m³	NIOSH RELs STEL/CEIL(C) ppm	NIOSH RELs STEL/CEIL(C) mg/m³	DFG MAKs TWA ppm	DFG MAKs TWA mg/m³	DFG MAKs PEAK/CEIL(C) ppm	DFG MAKs PEAK/CEIL(C) mg/m³	AIHA WEELs TWA ppm	AIHA WEELs TWA mg/m³	AIHA WEELs STEL/CEIL(C) ppm	AIHA WEELs STEL/CEIL(C) mg/m³	CARCINOGENICITY CATEGORY
Creosotes 8001-58-9																					EPA-B1 IARC-2A
Cresidine, m-isomer 102-50-1																					IARC-3
Cresidine, p-isomer (5-Methyl-o-anisidine) 120-71-8																					IARC-2B MAK-2 NTP-R
Cresol, all isomers 95-48-7; 106-44-5; 108-39-4; 1319-77-3		20 **IFV** Skin			5	22 Skin			2.3	10				Skin							EPA-C* MAK-3A TLV-A4 *o, m, p isomers only
Crotonaldehyde 4170-30-3; 123-73-9			C 0.3 Skin	C 0.86	2	6			2	6 *See* Pocket Guide App. C				Skin; 3B							EPA-C IARC-3 MAK-3B TLV-A3
Crufomate 299-86-5		5 BEI_A								5		20									TLV-A4
Cumene 98-82-8	50	246			50	245 Skin			50	245 Skin			10	50 Skin; C	II (4)						EPA-CBD; D IARC-2B MAK-3B
Cumene hydroperoxide 80-15-9																	1	6 Skin			EPA-C
Cupferron 135-20-6																					NTP-R

SUBSTANCE	ACGIH® TLVs®				OSHA PELs				NIOSH RELs				DFG MAKs				AIHA WEELs				CARCINOGENICITY CATEGORY
	TWA		STEL/CEIL(C)		TWA		STEL/CEIL(C)		TWA		STEL/CEIL(C)		TWA		PEAK/CEIL(C)		TWA		STEL/CEIL(C)		
CAS#	ppm	mg/m³	ppm	mg/m³	ppm	mg/m³	ppm	mg/m³	ppm	mg/m³	ppm	mg/m³	ppm	mg/m³	ppm	mg/m³	ppm	mg/m³	ppm	mg/m³	
Cyanamide 420-04-2		2								2			0.2* *can also be found as vapor Skin; Sh; C	0.35 **I**	II (1)						
Cyanides, as CN					5		Skin						2 **I**		II (1) Skin; C						
Cyanide, free 57-12-5																					EPA-D
Cyanogen 460-19-5	10	21							10	20			5	11	II (2) Skin; D						
Cyanogen chloride 506-77-4			C 0.3	C 0.75							C 0.3	C 0.6									
Cycasin 14901-08-7																					IARC-2B
Cyclochlorotine 12663-46-6																					IARC-3
Cyclohexane 110-82-7	100	344			300	1050			300	1050			200	700	II (4) D						EPA-I
Cyclohexanol 108-93-0	50	206	Skin		50	200			50	200	Skin										

SUBSTANCE / CAS#	ACGIH® TLVs® TWA ppm	ACGIH® TLVs® TWA mg/m³	ACGIH® TLVs® STEL/CEIL(C) ppm	ACGIH® TLVs® STEL/CEIL(C) mg/m³	OSHA PELs TWA ppm	OSHA PELs TWA mg/m³	OSHA PELs STEL/CEIL(C) ppm	OSHA PELs STEL/CEIL(C) mg/m³	NIOSH RELs TWA ppm	NIOSH RELs TWA mg/m³	NIOSH RELs STEL/CEIL(C) ppm	NIOSH RELs STEL/CEIL(C) mg/m³	DFG MAKs TWA ppm	DFG MAKs TWA mg/m³	DFG MAKs PEAK/CEIL(C) ppm	DFG MAKs PEAK/CEIL(C) mg/m³	AIHA WEELs TWA ppm	AIHA WEELs TWA mg/m³	AIHA WEELs STEL/CEIL(C) ppm	AIHA WEELs STEL/CEIL(C) mg/m³	CARCINOGENICITY CATEGORY
Cyclohexanone 108-94-1	20		50		50	200			25	100											IARC-3 MAK-3B TLV-A3
		Skin								Skin				Skin							
Cyclohexene 110-83-8	300	1010			300	1015			300	1015											
Cyclohexylamine 108-91-8	10	41							10	40			2	8.2	I (2)						TLV-A4
														C							
N-Cyclohexyl-2-benz-othiazolesulfenamide 95-33-0														Sh							
Cyclohexylhydroxydia-zene-1-oxide, potas-sium salt 66603-10-9													10 I		II (2)						
													Skin; D							
Cyclohexylmercaptan 1569-69-3											C 0.5*	C 2.4*								
										*15-min									
N-Cyclohexyl-N′-phen-yl-p-phenylenediamine 101-87-1														Sh							
Cyclonite (RDX) 121-82-4		0.5								1.5		3									EPA-C TLV-A4
		Skin								Skin										
4H-Cyclopenta[def]-chrysene 202-98-2																					IARC-3

SUBSTANCE CAS#	ACGIH® TLVs® TWA ppm	mg/m³	STEL/CEIL(C) ppm	mg/m³	OSHA PELs TWA ppm	mg/m³	STEL/CEIL(C) ppm	mg/m³	NIOSH RELs TWA ppm	mg/m³	STEL/CEIL(C) ppm	mg/m³	DFG MAKs TWA ppm	mg/m³	PEAK/CEIL(C)	AIHA WEELs TWA ppm	mg/m³	STEL/CEIL(C) ppm	mg/m³	CARCINOGENICITY CATEGORY
Cyclopentadiene 542-92-7	75	203			75	200			75	200										
Cyclopentane 287-92-3	600	1720							600	1720										
Cyclopenta[cd]pyrene 27208-37-3														Skin; 3B						IARC-2A MAK-2
5,6-Cyclopenteno-1,2-benzanthracene 7099-43-6																				IARC-3
Cyclophosphamide 50-18-0; 6055-19-2																				IARC-1 NTP-K* *CAS: 50-18-0
Cyclosporine 79217-60-0																				IARC-1
Cyclosporin A 59865-13-3																				NTP-K
Cyfluthrin 68359-37-5														0.01 I	I (1) C					
Cyhexatin (Tricyclohexyltin hydroxide) 13121-70-5		5				0.1* *as Sn				5										TLV-A4

SUBSTANCE / CAS#	ACGIH® TLVs® TWA ppm	ACGIH® TLVs® TWA mg/m³	ACGIH® TLVs® STEL/CEIL(C) ppm	ACGIH® TLVs® STEL/CEIL(C) mg/m³	OSHA PELs TWA ppm	OSHA PELs TWA mg/m³	OSHA PELs STEL/CEIL(C) ppm	OSHA PELs STEL/CEIL(C) mg/m³	NIOSH RELs TWA ppm	NIOSH RELs TWA mg/m³	NIOSH RELs STEL/CEIL(C) ppm	NIOSH RELs STEL/CEIL(C) mg/m³	DFG MAKs TWA ppm	DFG MAKs TWA mg/m³	DFG MAKs PEAK/CEIL(C) ppm	DFG MAKs PEAK/CEIL(C) mg/m³	AIHA WEELs TWA ppm	AIHA WEELs TWA mg/m³	AIHA WEELs STEL/CEIL(C) ppm	AIHA WEELs STEL/CEIL(C) mg/m³	CARCINOGENICITY CATEGORY
2,4-D (2,4-Dichloro-phenoxyacetic acid) 94-75-7		10 **I**				10				10				2 **I**		II (2)					TLV-A4
	Skin												including salts and esters Skin; C								
D and C Red No. 9 (Benzenesulfonic acid; 5-Chloro-2-[(2-hydroxy-1-naphthalenyl)azo]-4-methylbenzenesulfonic acid, barium salt (2:1)) 5160-02-1																		1			IARC-3
																as Barium salt (2:1)					
Dacarbazine 4342-03-4																					IARC-2B NTP-R
Dantron (Chrysazin; 1,8-Dihydroxyanthra-quinone) 117-10-2																					IARC-2B NTP-R
Dapsone 80-08-0																					IARC-3
Daunomycin 20830-81-3																					IARC-2B
Dawsonite, fibrous dust 12011-76-6																					MAK-2
DDT (Dichlorodiphenyl-trichloroethane) 50-29-3	1				1				0.5				1 **I**		II (8)						EPA-B2 TLV-A3 IARC-2B NIOSH-Ca NTP-R
						Skin			*See* Pocket Guide App. A					Skin							

| SUBSTANCE | ACGIH® TLVs® | | | | OSHA PELs | | | | NIOSH RELs | | | | DFG MAKs | | | | AIHA WEELs | | | | CARCINOGENICITY |
| | TWA | | STEL/CEIL(C) | | TWA | | STEL/CEIL(C) | | TWA | | STEL/CEIL(C) | | TWA | | PEAK/CEIL(C) | | TWA | | STEL/CEIL(C) | | |
CAS#	ppm	mg/m³	ppm	mg/m³	ppm	mg/m³	ppm	mg/m³	ppm	mg/m³	ppm	mg/m³	ppm	mg/m³	ppm	mg/m³	ppm	mg/m³	ppm	mg/m³	CATEGORY
Decaborane 17702-41-9	0.05	0.25	0.15	0.75	0.05	0.3			0.05	0.3	0.15	0.9	0.05	0.25	II (2)						
		Skin				Skin				Skin				Skin							
Decabromodiphenyl oxide 1163-19-5																		5			EPA-S IARC-3
1-Decene 872-05-9																	100				
Decylmercaptan 143-10-2											C 0.5*	C 3.6*									
										*15-min										
2-Dehydrolinalool 29171-20-8																	2				
Deltamethrin 52918-63-5																					IARC-3
Demeton 8065-48-3		0.05 IFV				0.1				0.1											
		Skin; BEI_A				Skin				Skin				Skin							
Demeton-S-methyl 919-86-8		0.05 IFV																			TLV-A4
	Skin; (SEN); BEI_A NIC-DSEN																				
Diacetone alcohol (4-Hydroxy-4-methyl-2-pentanone) 123-42-2	50	238			50	240			50	240			20	96	I (2)						
													Skin; D							

SUBSTANCE / CAS#	ACGIH® TLVs® TWA ppm	ACGIH® TLVs® TWA mg/m³	ACGIH® TLVs® STEL/CEIL(C) ppm	ACGIH® TLVs® STEL/CEIL(C) mg/m³	OSHA PELs TWA ppm	OSHA PELs TWA mg/m³	OSHA PELs STEL/CEIL(C) ppm	OSHA PELs STEL/CEIL(C) mg/m³	NIOSH RELs TWA ppm	NIOSH RELs TWA mg/m³	NIOSH RELs STEL/CEIL(C) ppm	NIOSH RELs STEL/CEIL(C) mg/m³	DFG MAKs TWA ppm	DFG MAKs TWA mg/m³	DFG MAKs PEAK/CEIL(C) ppm	DFG MAKs PEAK/CEIL(C) mg/m³	AIHA WEELs TWA ppm	AIHA WEELs TWA mg/m³	AIHA WEELs STEL/CEIL(C) ppm	AIHA WEELs STEL/CEIL(C) mg/m³	CARCINOGENICITY CATEGORY
Diacetyl / 431-03-8	0.01	0.04	0.02	0.07																	TLV-A4
Diacetylaminoazo-toluene / 83-63-6																					IARC-3
N,N′-Diacetylbenzidine / 613-35-4																					IARC-2B
Diallate / 2303-16-4																					IARC-3
Diallylamine / 124-02-7																	1		Skin		
2,4-Diaminoanisole / 615-05-4									and its salts; minimize occupational exposure (especially skin exposures) *See Pocket Guide App. A*					Skin							IARC-2B MAK-2 NIOSH-Ca
2,4-Diaminoanisole sulfate / 39156-41-7																					NTP-R
3,3′-Diaminobenzidine [91-95-2] and 3,3′-Dia-minobenzidine tetrahydrochloride [7411-49-6]																					MAK-3B

SUBSTANCE / CAS#	ACGIH® TLVs® TWA ppm	mg/m³	STEL/CEIL(C) ppm	mg/m³	OSHA PELs TWA ppm	mg/m³	STEL/CEIL(C) ppm	mg/m³	NIOSH RELs TWA ppm	mg/m³	STEL/CEIL(C) ppm	mg/m³	DFG MAKs TWA ppm	mg/m³	PEAK/CEIL(C)	AIHA WEELs TWA ppm	mg/m³	STEL/CEIL(C) ppm	mg/m³	CARCINOGENICITY CATEGORY
1,2-Diamino-4-nitro-benzene 99-56-9																				IARC-3
2,4-Diaminotoluene (Toluene-2,4-diamine) 95-80-7									all isomers See Pocket Guide App. A						Skin; Sh	0.005 and mixed isomers CAS: 25376-45-8 Skin				IARC-2B MAK-2 NIOSH-Ca NTP-R
2,5-Diaminotoluene (Toluene-2,5-diamine) 95-70-5															Sh					IARC-3
Dianisidine-based dyes									minimize exposure; handle with caution See Pocket Guide App. C											NIOSH-Ca
Diazepam 439-14-5																				IARC-3
Diazinon 333-41-5	0.01 **IFV** Skin; BEI_A								0.1 Skin				0.1 **I** Skin; C		**II** (2)					TLV-A4
Diazoaminobenzene 136-35-6																				NTP-R
Diazomethane 334-88-3	0.2	0.34			0.2	0.4			0.2	0.4										IARC-3 MAK-2 TLV-A2
Dibenz[a,h]acridine 226-36-8																				IARC-2B NTP-R

SUBSTANCE / CAS#	ACGIH® TLVs® TWA ppm	ACGIH® TLVs® TWA mg/m³	ACGIH® TLVs® STEL/CEIL(C) ppm	ACGIH® TLVs® STEL/CEIL(C) mg/m³	OSHA PELs TWA ppm	OSHA PELs TWA mg/m³	OSHA PELs STEL/CEIL(C) ppm	OSHA PELs STEL/CEIL(C) mg/m³	NIOSH RELs TWA ppm	NIOSH RELs TWA mg/m³	NIOSH RELs STEL/CEIL(C) ppm	NIOSH RELs STEL/CEIL(C) mg/m³	DFG MAKs TWA ppm	DFG MAKs TWA mg/m³	DFG MAKs PEAK/CEIL(C) ppm	DFG MAKs PEAK/CEIL(C) mg/m³	AIHA WEELs TWA ppm	AIHA WEELs TWA mg/m³	AIHA WEELs STEL/CEIL(C) ppm	AIHA WEELs STEL/CEIL(C) mg/m³	CARCINOGENICITY CATEGORY
Dibenz[a,j]acridine 224-42-0																					IARC-2A NTP-R
Dibenz[c,h]acridine 224-53-3																					IARC-2B
Dibenz[a,c]anthracene 215-58-7																					IARC-3
Dibenz[a,h]anthracene 53-70-3														Skin; 3A							EPA-B2 IARC-2A MAK-2 NTP-R
Dibenz[a,j]anthracene 224-41-9																					IARC-3
7H-Dibenzo[c,g]-carbazole 194-59-2																					IARC-2B NTP-R
Dibenzo-p-dioxin 262-12-4																					IARC-3
Dibenzo[a,e]fluoran-thene 5385-75-1																					IARC-3
13H-Dibenzo[a,g]-fluorene 207-83-0																					IARC-3

SUBSTANCE CAS#	ACGIH® TLVs® TWA		STEL/CEIL(C)		OSHA PELs TWA		STEL/CEIL(C)		NIOSH RELs TWA		STEL/CEIL(C)		DFG MAKs TWA		PEAK/CEIL(C)	AIHA WEELs TWA		STEL/CEIL(C)		CARCINOGENICITY CATEGORY
	ppm	mg/m³	ppm	mg/m³	ppm	mg/m³	ppm	mg/m³	ppm	mg/m³	ppm	mg/m³	ppm	mg/m³		ppm	mg/m³	ppm	mg/m³	
Dibenzofuran 132-64-9																				EPA-D
Dibenzo[h,rst]penta-phene 192-47-2																				IARC-3
Dibenzo[a,e]pyrene 192-65-4															Skin; 3B					IARC-3 MAK-2 NTP-R
Dibenzo[a,h]pyrene 189-64-0															Skin; 3B					IARC-2B MAK-2 NTP-R
Dibenzo[a,i]pyrene 189-55-9															Skin; 3B					IARC-2B MAK-2 NTP-R
Dibenzo[a,l]pyrene 191-30-0															Skin; 3B					IARC-2A MAK-2 NTP-R
Dibenzo[e,l]pyrene 192-51-8																				IARC-3
2,2´-Dibenzothiazyl disulfide 120-78-5															Sh					
Dibenzothiopene 132-65-0																				IARC-3

SUBSTANCE / CAS#	ACGIH® TLVs® TWA ppm	mg/m³	STEL/CEIL(C) ppm	mg/m³	OSHA PELs TWA ppm	mg/m³	STEL/CEIL(C) ppm	mg/m³	NIOSH RELs TWA ppm	mg/m³	STEL/CEIL(C) ppm	mg/m³	DFG MAKs TWA ppm	mg/m³	PEAK/CEIL(C) ppm	mg/m³	AIHA WEELs TWA ppm	mg/m³	STEL/CEIL(C) ppm	mg/m³	CARCINOGENICITY CATEGORY
Diborane 19287-45-7	0.1	0.11			0.1	0.1			0.1	0.1											
Dibromoacetic acid 631-64-1																					IARC-2B
Dibromoacetonitrile 3252-43-5																					IARC-2B
1,2-Dibromo-3-chloro- propane (DBCP) 96-12-8					0.001																IARC-2B OSHA-Ca MAK-2 NIOSH-Ca NTP-R
					See 29 CFR 1910.1044				See Pocket Guide App. A				Skin; 2								
2,2-Dibromo-2-cyan- acetamide 10222-01-2													Sh								
Dibromodichloro- methane 594-18-3																					EPA-D
1,2-Dibromo-2,4- dicyanobutane 35691-65-7													Sh								
p,p′-Dibromodiphenyl ether 2050-47-7																					EPA-D
2,3-Dibromo-1-propanol 96-13-9																					IARC-2B NTP-R

SUBSTANCE / CAS#	ACGIH® TLVs®				OSHA PELs				NIOSH RELs				DFG MAKs			AIHA WEELs				CARCINOGENICITY CATEGORY
	TWA		STEL/CEIL(C)		TWA		STEL/CEIL(C)		TWA		STEL/CEIL(C)		TWA		PEAK/CEIL(C)	TWA		STEL/CEIL(C)		
	ppm	mg/m³	ppm	mg/m³	ppm	mg/m³	ppm	mg/m³	ppm	mg/m³	ppm	mg/m³	ppm	mg/m³		ppm	mg/m³	ppm	mg/m³	
tris(2,3-Dibromopropyl)-phosphate 126-72-7																				IARC-2A NTP-R
Dibutylamine 111-92-2																	Skin	C 5		
2-N-Dibutylaminoethanol 102-81-8	0.5	3.5							2	14										
		Skin; BEI$_A$								Skin										
Dibutyl phenyl phosphate 2528-36-1	0.3	3.5																		
		Skin; BEI$_A$																		
Dibutyl phosphate 107-66-4	0.6 IFV	5 IFV			1	5			1	5	2	10								MAK-3A
		Skin																		
Dibutyl phthalate 84-74-2		5				5				5			0.05	0.58	I (2)					EPA-D MAK-4
													C						
Di-n-butyltin compounds, as Sn													0.004*	0.02 I	I (1)					MAK-4
													Skin**; B						
												*can also be found as vapor							
												**for n-butyltin cmpds whose organic ligands were already designated "Sa" or "Sh", these designations also apply							
Dicarboxylic acid (C$_4$–C$_6$) dimethyl ester, mixture 95481-62-2													0.75	5	I (1)					
													C						

SUBSTANCE / CAS#	ACGIH® TLVs® TWA ppm	mg/m³	STEL/CEIL(C) ppm	mg/m³	OSHA PELs TWA ppm	mg/m³	STEL/CEIL(C) ppm	mg/m³	NIOSH RELs TWA ppm	mg/m³	STEL/CEIL(C) ppm	mg/m³	DFG MAKs TWA ppm	mg/m³	PEAK/CEIL(C) ppm	mg/m³	AIHA WEELs TWA ppm	mg/m³	STEL/CEIL(C) ppm	mg/m³	CARCINOGENICITY CATEGORY
Dichloroacetic acid 79-43-6	0.5	2.64																			EPA-L IARC-2B MAK-3A TLV-A3
		Skin																			
Dichloroacetonitrile 3018-12-0																					IARC-3
Dichloroacetylene 7572-29-4			C 0.1	C 0.39							C 0.1	C 0.4									IARC-3 MAK-2 NIOSH-Ca TLV-A3
									See Pocket Guide App. A												
3,4-Dichloroaniline 95-76-1															Skin; Sh						
Dichlorobenzene, m-isomer 541-73-1													2	12	II (2)						EPA-D IARC-3
														C						
Dichlorobenzene, o-isomer (1,2-Dichlorobenzene) 95-50-1	25	150	50	301			C 50	C 300			C 50	C 300	10	61	II (2)						EPA-D IARC-3 TLV-A4
														Skin; C						
Dichlorobenzene, p-isomer (1,4-Dichlorobenzene) 106-46-7	10	60			75	450									Skin; 3B						IARC-2B NTP-R MAK-2 TLV-A3 NIOSH-Ca
									See Pocket Guide App. A												
3,3'-Dichlorobenzidine 91-94-1										and its salts					Skin						EPA-B2 NTP-R IARC-2B OSHA-Ca MAK-2 TLV-A3 NIOSH-Ca
		Skin; L			_See_ 29 CFR 1910.1003				_See_ Pocket Guide App. A												
3,3'-Dichlorobenzidine dihydrochloride 612-83-9																					NTP-R

SUBSTANCE / CAS#	ACGIH® TLVs® TWA ppm	mg/m³	STEL/CEIL(C) ppm	mg/m³	OSHA PELs TWA ppm	mg/m³	STEL/CEIL(C) ppm	mg/m³	NIOSH RELs TWA ppm	mg/m³	STEL/CEIL(C) ppm	mg/m³	DFG MAKs TWA ppm	mg/m³	PEAK/CEIL(C) ppm	mg/m³	AIHA WEELs TWA ppm	mg/m³	STEL/CEIL(C) ppm	mg/m³	CARCINOGENICITY CATEGORY
1,4-Dichloro-2-butene 764-41-0	0.005	0.025																			MAK-2 TLV-A2
		Skin												Skin; 3A							
1,4-Dichlorobutene, trans-isomer 110-57-6																					IARC-3
3,3′-Dichloro-4,4′-di-aminodiphenyl ether 28434-86-8																					IARC-2B
Dichlorodifluoromethane (FC-12) 75-71-8	1000	4950			1000	4950			1000	4950			1000	5000	II (2) C						TLV-A4
1,3-Dichloro-5,5-dimethyl hydantoin 118-52-5		0.2		0.4		0.2				0.2		0.4									
p,p′-Dichlorodiphenyl-dichloroethane (DDD) 72-54-8																					EPA-B2
p,p′-Dichlorodiphenyl-dichloroethylene (DDE) 72-55-9																					EPA-B2
1,1-Dichloroethane (Ethylidene chloride) 75-34-3	100	405			100	400			100	400 *See* Pocket Guide App. C			100	410	II (2) C						EPA-C TLV-A4
1,2-Dichloroethylene, all isomers (Acetylene dichloride) 156-59-2; 156-60-5; 540-59-0	200	793			200	790			200	790			200	800	II (2)						EPA-II* *CAS: 156-59-2; 156-60-5

SUBSTANCE CAS#	ACGIH® TLVs® TWA ppm	ACGIH® TLVs® TWA mg/m³	ACGIH® TLVs® STEL/CEIL(C) ppm	ACGIH® TLVs® STEL/CEIL(C) mg/m³	OSHA PELs TWA ppm	OSHA PELs TWA mg/m³	OSHA PELs STEL/CEIL(C) ppm	OSHA PELs STEL/CEIL(C) mg/m³	NIOSH RELs TWA ppm	NIOSH RELs TWA mg/m³	NIOSH RELs STEL/CEIL(C) ppm	NIOSH RELs STEL/CEIL(C) mg/m³	DFG MAKs TWA ppm	DFG MAKs TWA mg/m³	DFG MAKs PEAK/CEIL(C) ppm	DFG MAKs PEAK/CEIL(C) mg/m³	AIHA WEELs TWA ppm	AIHA WEELs TWA mg/m³	AIHA WEELs STEL/CEIL(C) ppm	AIHA WEELs STEL/CEIL(C) mg/m³	CARCINOGENICITY CATEGORY
Dichloroethyl ether (bis[2-Chloroethyl]ether) 111-44-4	5	29	10	58 Skin			C 15	C 90 Skin	5	30	10 Skin See Pocket Guide App. A	60	10	59	I (1)	Skin					EPA-B2 IARC-3 NIOSH-Ca TLV-A4
1,1-Dichloro-1-fluoro-ethane 1717-00-6																	500	2370	3000* *5 min	14,220*	
Dichlorofluoromethane (FC-21) 75-43-4	10	42			1000	4200			10	40			10	43	II (2)						
Dichloromethane (Methylene chloride) 75-09-2	50	174		BEI	25			125 See 29 CFR 1910.1052			See Pocket Guide App. A										EPA-L NTP-R IARC-2B OSHA-Ca MAK-3A TLV-A3 NIOSH-Ca
1,2-Dichloromethoxy-ethane 41683-62-9															Skin						MAK-3B
3,4-Dichloronitroben-zene 99-54-7															Skin		1				MAK-3B
1,1-Dichloro-1-nitro-ethane 594-72-9	2	12					C 10	C 60	2	10											
2,4-Dichlorophenol 120-83-2															Skin; Q		1				IARC-2B
4-(2,4-Dichlorophenoxy)-benzenamine 14861-17-7															Skin						MAK-3B

SUBSTANCE CAS#	ACGIH® TLVs TWA ppm	mg/m³	STEL/CEIL(C) ppm	mg/m³	OSHA PELs TWA ppm	mg/m³	STEL/CEIL(C) ppm	mg/m³	NIOSH RELs TWA ppm	mg/m³	STEL/CEIL(C) ppm	mg/m³	DFG MAKs TWA ppm	mg/m³	PEAK/CEIL(C) ppm	mg/m³	AIHA WEELs TWA ppm	mg/m³	STEL/CEIL(C) ppm	mg/m³	CARCINOGENICITY CATEGORY
2,6-Dichloro-p-phenyl-enediamine 609-20-1																					IARC-3
1,3-Dichloro-2-propanol 96-23-1														Skin							IARC-2B MAK-2
1,3-Dichloropropene 542-75-6	1	4.5 Skin							1	5 Skin See Pocket Guide App. A			cis- and trans-isomers Skin; Sh								EPA-B2; K NIOSH-Ca IARC-2B* NTP-R* MAK-2 TLV-A3 *technical grade
2,2-Dichloropropionic acid 75-99-0	5 I								1	6											TLV-A4
Dichlorotetrafluoroethane (1,2-Dichloro-1,1,2,2-tetrafluoroethane) 76-14-2	1000	6990			1000	7000			1000	7000			1000	7100	II (8) D						TLV-A4
2,2-Dichloro-1,1,1-tri-fluoroethane (FC-123) 306-83-2																	50				MAK-3B
Dichlorvos (DDVP) 62-73-7	0.1 IFV Skin; (SEN); BEIₐ NIC-DSEN				1 Skin				1 Skin				0.11 Skin; C	1	II (2)						EPA-B2 IARC-2B TLV-A4
Dicofol 115-32-2																					IARC-3
Dicrotophos 141-66-2	0.05 IFV Skin; BEIₐ								0.25 Skin												TLV-A4

SUBSTANCE CAS#	ACGIH® TLVs® TWA ppm	TWA mg/m³	STEL/CEIL(C) ppm	STEL/CEIL(C) mg/m³	OSHA PELs TWA ppm	TWA mg/m³	STEL/CEIL(C) ppm	STEL/CEIL(C) mg/m³	NIOSH RELs TWA ppm	TWA mg/m³	STEL/CEIL(C) ppm	STEL/CEIL(C) mg/m³	DFG MAKs TWA ppm	TWA mg/m³	PEAK/CEIL(C) ppm	PEAK/CEIL(C) mg/m³	AIHA WEELs TWA ppm	TWA mg/m³	STEL/CEIL(C) ppm	STEL/CEIL(C) mg/m³	CARCINOGENICITY CATEGORY
Dicyclohexylamine 101-83-7														Skin							
1,3-Dicyclohexyl-carbodiimide 538-75-0														Sh							
Dicyclopentadiene 77-73-6	5	27							5	30			0.5	2.7	I (1) D						
Dicyclopentadienyl iron, as Fe (Ferrocene) 102-54-5		10			15*; 5** *Total dust **Respirable fraction				10*; 5** *Total dust **Respirable fraction												
Didanosine 69655-05-6																					IARC-3
Di(tert-dodecyl) penta-sulfide 31565-23-8														100 I C	II (2)						
Di(tert-dodecyl) poly-sulfides 68425-15-0; 68583-56-2														100 I C	II (2)						
Dieldrin 60-57-1		0.1 IFV Skin				0.25 Skin				0.25 Skin *See* Pocket Guide App. A				0.25 I Skin	II (8)						EPA-B2 IARC-3 NIOSH-Ca TLV-A3
Diepoxybutane 1464-53-5														2							IARC-2A NTP-R

SUBSTANCE / CAS#	ACGIH® TLVs® TWA ppm	TWA mg/m³	STEL/CEIL(C) ppm	STEL/CEIL(C) mg/m³	OSHA PELs TWA ppm	TWA mg/m³	STEL/CEIL(C) ppm	STEL/CEIL(C) mg/m³	NIOSH RELs TWA ppm	TWA mg/m³	STEL/CEIL(C) ppm	STEL/CEIL(C) mg/m³	DFG MAKs TWA ppm	TWA mg/m³	PEAK/CEIL(C) ppm	PEAK/CEIL(C) mg/m³	AIHA WEELs TWA ppm	TWA mg/m³	STEL/CEIL(C) ppm	STEL/CEIL(C) mg/m³	CARCINOGENICITY CATEGORY
Diesel engine emissions								See Pocket Guide App. A													EPA-L NTP-R IARC-2A MAK-2 NIOSH-Ca
Diesel fuel 68334-30-5; 68476-30-2; 68476-34-6; 77650-28-3	100 **IFV** as total hydrocarbons Skin																				IARC-2B TLV-A3
Diesel fuels, distillate (light)																					IARC-3
Diethanolamine 111-42-2	0.2 **IFV**	1 **IFV** Skin							3	15			1 I		I (1) Skin; Sh; C						IARC-2B MAK-3B TLV-A3
Diethylamine 109-89-7	5	15 Skin	15	45	25	75			10	30	25	75	5	15	I (2) C 10 C 30 D						TLV-A4
2-Diethylaminoethanol 100-37-8	2	9.6 Skin			10	50 Skin			10	50 Skin			5	24	I (1) Skin; C						
Diethylbenzene, mixed isomers 25340-17-4																	5				
Diethylcarbamoyl chloride 88-10-8																					MAK-3B
Diethylene glycol 111-46-6													10	44	II (4) C		10				

SUBSTANCE / CAS#	ACGIH® TLVs® TWA ppm	mg/m³	STEL/CEIL(C) ppm	mg/m³	OSHA PELs TWA ppm	mg/m³	STEL/CEIL(C) ppm	mg/m³	NIOSH RELs TWA ppm	mg/m³	STEL/CEIL(C) ppm	mg/m³	DFG MAKs TWA ppm	mg/m³	PEAK/CEIL(C) ppm	mg/m³	AIHA WEELs TWA ppm	mg/m³	STEL/CEIL(C) ppm	mg/m³	CARCINOGENICITY CATEGORY
Diethylene glycol diacrylate 4074-88-8															Sh						
Diethylene glycol dimethacrylate 2358-84-1															Sh						
Diethylene glycol dimethyl ether 111-96-6													5	28	II (8)						
													Skin; B								
Diethylene glycol dinitrate 693-21-0															Skin						EPA-D
Diethylene glycol monobutyl ether 112-34-5	10*	67.5*											10*	67	I (1.5)						
	*IFV												*sum of the concentrations of DGBE and its acetate in air C								
Diethylene triamine 111-40-0	1	4.2							1	4					Sh						
		Skin								Skin											
Di(2-ethylhexyl)adipate 103-23-1																					EPA-C IARC-3
Di(2-ethylhexyl)phthalate (DEHP) 117-81-7		5				5				5		10		10	II (8)						EPA-B2 NIOSH-Ca IARC-2B NTP-R MAK-4 TLV-A3
					See Pocket Guide App. A								C								
1,2-Diethylhydrazine 1615-80-1																					IARC-2B

SUBSTANCE / CAS#	ACGIH® TLVs® TWA ppm	mg/m³	STEL/CEIL(C) ppm	mg/m³	OSHA PELs TWA ppm	mg/m³	STEL/CEIL(C) ppm	mg/m³	NIOSH RELs TWA ppm	mg/m³	STEL/CEIL(C) ppm	mg/m³	DFG MAKs TWA ppm	mg/m³	PEAK/CEIL(C) ppm	mg/m³	AIHA WEELs TWA ppm	mg/m³	STEL/CEIL(C) ppm	mg/m³	CARCINOGENICITY CATEGORY
N,N-Diethylhydroxyla-mine 3710-84-7	2	7.3																			
Diethyl ketone 96-22-0	200	705	300	1057					200	705											
Diethyl-p-nitrophenyl-phosphate 311-45-5																					EPA-D
Diethyl phthalate 84-66-2		5								5											EPA-D TLV-A4
Diethylstilboestrol 56-53-1																					IARC-1 NTP-K
Diethyl sulfate 64-67-5														Skin; 2							IARC-2A MAK-2 NTP-R
N,N′-Diethylthiourea 105-55-5																					IARC-3
Difluorodibromo-methane 75-61-6	100	858			100	860			100	860											
1,1-Difluoroethane 75-37-6																	1000				

SUBSTANCE / CAS#	ACGIH® TLVs® TWA ppm	ACGIH® TLVs® TWA mg/m³	ACGIH® TLVs® STEL/CEIL(C) ppm	ACGIH® TLVs® STEL/CEIL(C) mg/m³	OSHA PELs TWA ppm	OSHA PELs TWA mg/m³	OSHA PELs STEL/CEIL(C) ppm	OSHA PELs STEL/CEIL(C) mg/m³	NIOSH RELs TWA ppm	NIOSH RELs TWA mg/m³	NIOSH RELs STEL/CEIL(C) ppm	NIOSH RELs STEL/CEIL(C) mg/m³	DFG MAKs TWA ppm	DFG MAKs TWA mg/m³	DFG MAKs PEAK/CEIL(C) ppm	DFG MAKs PEAK/CEIL(C) mg/m³	AIHA WEELs TWA ppm	AIHA WEELs TWA mg/m³	AIHA WEELs STEL/CEIL(C) ppm	AIHA WEELs STEL/CEIL(C) mg/m³	CARCINOGENICITY CATEGORY
Difluoromethane 75-10-5																	1000				
Diglycidyl ether (DGE) 2238-07-5	0.01	0.05					C 0.5	C 2.8	0.1	0.5											MAK-3B NIOSH-Ca TLV-A4
						See Pocket Guide App. A							Skin								
Diglycidyl hexanediol 16096-31-4														Sh							
Diglycidyl resorcinol ether 101-90-6														Skin; Sh							IARC-2B MAK-2 NTP-R
1,2-Dihydroacean-thrylene 641-48-5																					IARC-3
Dihydrosafrole 94-58-6																					IARC-2B
Dihydroxymethyl-furatrizine 794-93-4																					IARC-3
Diisobutylene 107-39-1																	75				
Diisobutyl ketone (2,6-Dimethyl-4-heptanone) 108-83-8	25	145			50	290			25	150											

SUBSTANCE CAS#	ACGIH® TLVs® TWA ppm	ACGIH® TLVs® TWA mg/m³	ACGIH® TLVs® STEL/CEIL(C) ppm	ACGIH® TLVs® STEL/CEIL(C) mg/m³	OSHA PELs TWA ppm	OSHA PELs TWA mg/m³	OSHA PELs STEL/CEIL(C) ppm	OSHA PELs STEL/CEIL(C) mg/m³	NIOSH RELs TWA ppm	NIOSH RELs TWA mg/m³	NIOSH RELs STEL/CEIL(C) ppm	NIOSH RELs STEL/CEIL(C) mg/m³	DFG MAKs TWA ppm	DFG MAKs TWA mg/m³	DFG MAKs PEAK/CEIL(C) ppm	DFG MAKs PEAK/CEIL(C) mg/m³	AIHA WEELs TWA ppm	AIHA WEELs TWA mg/m³	AIHA WEELs STEL/CEIL(C) ppm	AIHA WEELs STEL/CEIL(C) mg/m³	CARCINOGENICITY CATEGORY
Diisodecyl phthalate 26761-40-0																					MAK-3B
Diisopropylamine 108-18-9	5	21		Skin	5	20		Skin	5	20		Skin									
Diisopropyl methyl-phosphonate (DIMP) 1445-75-6																					EPA-D
Diisopropyl sulfate 2973-10-6																					IARC-2B
Dimethipin 55290-64-7																					EPA-C
Dimethoxane 828-00-2																					IARC-3
3,3'-Dimethoxybenzidine (o-Dianisidine-based dyes) 119-90-4									*See* Pocket Guide Apps. A and C												IARC-2B MAK-2 NIOSH-Ca NTP-R
3,3'-Dimethoxybenzidine [119-90-4], dyes metabolized to this compound																					NTP-R
3,3'-Dimethoxybenzidine-4,4'-diisocyanate 91-93-0																					IARC-3

SUBSTANCE / CAS#	ACGIH® TLVs® TWA ppm	mg/m³	STEL/CEIL(C) ppm	mg/m³	OSHA PELs TWA ppm	mg/m³	STEL/CEIL(C) ppm	mg/m³	NIOSH RELs TWA ppm	mg/m³	STEL/CEIL(C) ppm	mg/m³	DFG MAKs TWA ppm	mg/m³	PEAK/CEIL(C) ppm	mg/m³	AIHA WEELs TWA ppm	mg/m³	STEL/CEIL(C) ppm	mg/m³	CARCINOGENICITY CATEGORY
2,5-Dimethoxy-4-chloroaniline 6358-64-1													Skin								MAK-3B
N,N-Dimethylacetamide 127-19-5	10	36			10	35			10	35			10	36	II (2)						TLV-A4
	Skin; BEI				Skin				Skin				Skin; C								
Dimethylamine 124-40-3	5	9.2	15	27.6	10	18			10	18			2	3.7	I (2)		1		3		TLV-A4
	NIC-DSEN													D							
4-Dimethylaminoazo-benzene 60-11-7					See 29 CFR 1910.1003				See Pocket Guide App. A												IARC-2B NIOSH-Ca NTP-R OSHA-Ca
p-Dimethylaminoazo-benzenediazo sodium sulfonate 140-56-7																					IARC-3
bis(2-Dimethylamino-ethyl) ether (DMAEE) 3033-62-3	0.05	0.33	0.15	0.98					minimize exposure See also NIAX® Catalyst ESN See Pocket Guide App. C												
	Skin																				
trans-2-[(Dimethyl-amino)methylimino]-5-[2-(5-nitro-2-furyl)-vinyl]-1,3,4-oxadiazole 25962-77-0																					IARC-2B
Dimethylaminopro-pionitrile 1738-25-6									minimize exposure See also NIAX® Catalyst ESN See Pocket Guide App. C												

SUBSTANCE / CAS#	ACGIH® TLVs® TWA ppm	mg/m³	STEL/CEIL(C) ppm	mg/m³	OSHA PELs TWA ppm	mg/m³	STEL/CEIL(C) ppm	mg/m³	NIOSH RELs TWA ppm	mg/m³	STEL/CEIL(C) ppm	mg/m³	DFG MAKs TWA ppm	mg/m³	PEAK/CEIL(C) ppm	mg/m³	AIHA WEELs TWA ppm	mg/m³	STEL/CEIL(C) ppm	mg/m³	CARCINOGENICITY CATEGORY
4,4′-Dimethylangelicin plus ultraviolet A radiation 22975-76-4																					IARC-3
4,5′-Dimethylangelicin plus ultraviolet A radiation 4063-41-6																					IARC-3
Dimethylaniline (N,N-Dimethylaniline) 121-69-7	5	25	10	50	5	25			5	25	10	50	5	25	II (2)						IARC-3 MAK-3B TLV-A4
	Skin; BEI$_M$				Skin				Skin				Skin; D								
N-(1,3-Dimethyl butyl)-N′-phenyl-p-phenylene-diamine 793-24-8													2 I		II (2)						
													Sh; C								
Dimethyl carbamoyl chloride 79-44-7	0.005	0.02																			IARC-2A TLV-A2 MAK-2 NIOSH-Ca NTP-R
	Skin				See Pocket Guide App. A								Skin								
Dimethyldichlorosilane 75-78-5																			C 2		
Dimethyl disulfide 624-92-0	0.5	2																			
	Skin																				
Dimethyl ether 115-10-6													1000	1900	II (8)		1000				
													D								
Dimethylethoxysilane 14857-34-2	0.5	2.1	1.5	6.4																	

SUBSTANCE CAS#	ACGIH® TLVs® TWA ppm	ACGIH® TLVs® TWA mg/m³	STEL/CEIL(C) ppm	STEL/CEIL(C) mg/m³	OSHA PELs TWA ppm	OSHA PELs TWA mg/m³	STEL/CEIL(C) ppm	STEL/CEIL(C) mg/m³	NIOSH RELs TWA ppm	NIOSH RELs TWA mg/m³	STEL/CEIL(C) ppm	STEL/CEIL(C) mg/m³	DFG MAKs TWA ppm	DFG MAKs TWA mg/m³	PEAK/CEIL(C) ppm	PEAK/CEIL(C) mg/m³	AIHA WEELs TWA ppm	AIHA WEELs TWA mg/m³	STEL/CEIL(C) ppm	STEL/CEIL(C) mg/m³	CARCINOGENICITY CATEGORY
N,N-Dimethylethyl-amine 598-56-1													2	6.1	I (2) D						
Dimethylformamide 68-12-2	10	30 Skin; BEI			10	30 Skin			10	30 Skin			5	15 Skin; B	II (2)						IARC-3 TLV-A4
1,1-Dimethylhydrazine 57-14-7	0.01	0.025 Skin			0.5	1 Skin					C 0.06* See Pocket Guide App. A	C 0.15* *120-min		Skin; Sh							IARC-2B MAK-2 NIOSH-Ca NTP-R TLV-A3
1,2-Dimethylhydrazine 540-73-8														Skin; Sh							IARC-2A MAK-2
Dimethyl hydrogen phosphite 868-85-9																					IARC-3 MAK-3B
N,N-Dimethylisopropyl-amine 996-35-0													1	3.6	I (2) D						
Dimethyloldihydroxy-ethylene urea 1854-26-8														Sh							
1,3-Dimethylol-5,5-di-methyl hydantoin 6440-58-0														Sh							
1,4-Dimethylphenan-threne 22349-59-3																					IARC-3

SUBSTANCE / CAS#	ACGIH® TLVs® TWA ppm	TWA mg/m³	STEL/CEIL(C) ppm	mg/m³	OSHA PELs TWA ppm	TWA mg/m³	STEL/CEIL(C) ppm	mg/m³	NIOSH RELs TWA ppm	TWA mg/m³	STEL/CEIL(C) ppm	mg/m³	DFG MAKs TWA ppm	TWA mg/m³	PEAK/CEIL(C)	AIHA WEELs TWA ppm	TWA mg/m³	STEL/CEIL(C) ppm	mg/m³	CARCINOGENICITY CATEGORY
Dimethylphthalate 131-11-3		5				5				5										EPA-D
N,N-Dimethyl-p-tolui-dine 99-97-8																0.5				
Dimethylsulfamoyl chloride 13360-57-1														Skin						MAK-2
Dimethyl sulfate 77-78-1	0.1	0.52			1	5			0.1	0.5										EPA-B2 NTP-R IARC-2A TLV-A3 MAK-2 NIOSH-Ca
	Skin				Skin				Skin *See* Pocket Guide App. A				Skin							
Dimethyl sulfide 75-18-3	10	25																		
Dimethyl sulfoxide 67-68-5													50	160	I (2)	250				
													Skin; D						
Dimethyl terephthalate 120-61-6																	5*			
															*Total dust				
Dinitrobenzene, all isomers 99-65-0; 100-25-4; 528-29-0; 25154-54-5	0.15	1				1				1										EPA-D* MAK-3B *o-, m-isomers
	Skin; BEI_M				Skin				Skin				Skin							
3,7-Dinitrofluoranthene 105735-71-5																				IARC-2B

SUBSTANCE / CAS#	ACGIH® TLVs® TWA ppm	TWA mg/m³	STEL/CEIL(C) ppm	STEL/CEIL(C) mg/m³	OSHA PELs TWA ppm	TWA mg/m³	STEL/CEIL(C) ppm	STEL/CEIL(C) mg/m³	NIOSH RELs TWA ppm	TWA mg/m³	STEL/CEIL(C) ppm	STEL/CEIL(C) mg/m³	DFG MAKs TWA ppm	TWA mg/m³	PEAK/CEIL(C) ppm	PEAK/CEIL(C) mg/m³	AIHA WEELs TWA ppm	TWA mg/m³	STEL/CEIL(C) ppm	STEL/CEIL(C) mg/m³	CARCINOGENICITY CATEGORY
3,9-Dinitrofluoranthene 22506-53-2																					IARC-2B
4,6-Dinitro-o-cresol 534-52-1		0.2 Skin				0.2 Skin				0.2 Skin				Skin							
Dinitronaphthalene, all isomers 27478-34-8																					MAK-3B
1,3-Dinitropyrene 75321-20-9																					IARC-2B
1,6-Dinitropyrene 42397-64-8																					IARC-2B NTP-R
1,8-Dinitropyrene 42397-65-9																					IARC-2B NTP-R
3,5-Dinitro-o-toluamide (Dinitolmide) 148-01-6	1								5												TLV-A4
Dinitrosopentamethylenetetramine 101-25-7																					IARC-3
Dinitrotoluene 25321-14-6		0.2 Skin; BEI_M				1.5 Skin				1.5 Skin *See* Pocket Guide App. A				mixture of isomers Skin							EPA-B2* NIOSH-Ca MAK-2* TLV-A3 *mixture of isomers

SUBSTANCE CAS#	ACGIH® TLVs® TWA ppm	ACGIH® TLVs® TWA mg/m³	ACGIH® TLVs® STEL/CEIL(C) ppm	ACGIH® TLVs® STEL/CEIL(C) mg/m³	OSHA PELs TWA ppm	OSHA PELs TWA mg/m³	OSHA PELs STEL/CEIL(C) ppm	OSHA PELs STEL/CEIL(C) mg/m³	NIOSH RELs TWA ppm	NIOSH RELs TWA mg/m³	NIOSH RELs STEL/CEIL(C) ppm	NIOSH RELs STEL/CEIL(C) mg/m³	DFG MAKs TWA ppm	DFG MAKs TWA mg/m³	DFG MAKs PEAK/CEIL(C) ppm	DFG MAKs PEAK/CEIL(C) mg/m³	AIHA WEELs TWA ppm	AIHA WEELs TWA mg/m³	AIHA WEELs STEL/CEIL(C) ppm	AIHA WEELs STEL/CEIL(C) mg/m³	CARCINOGENICITY CATEGORY
2,4-Dinitrotoluene 121-14-2																					IARC-2B
2,6-Dinitrotoluene 606-20-2																					IARC-2B
3,5-Dinitrotoluene 618-85-9																					IARC-3
Dinoseb 88-85-7																					EPA-D
Di-n-octyltin compounds, as Sn													0.002*	0.0098 I		II (2) Skin**; B					MAK-4

*can also be found as vapor
**for n-octyltin cmpds whose organic ligands are already designated "Sa" or "Sh", these designations also apply

SUBSTANCE CAS#	ACGIH TWA ppm	ACGIH TWA mg/m³	ACGIH STEL ppm	ACGIH STEL mg/m³	OSHA TWA ppm	OSHA TWA mg/m³	OSHA STEL ppm	OSHA STEL mg/m³	NIOSH TWA ppm	NIOSH TWA mg/m³	NIOSH STEL ppm	NIOSH STEL mg/m³	DFG TWA ppm	DFG TWA mg/m³	DFG PEAK ppm	DFG PEAK mg/m³	AIHA TWA ppm	AIHA TWA mg/m³	AIHA STEL ppm	AIHA STEL mg/m³	CARC
1,4-Dioxane (Diethylene dioxide) 123-91-1	20	72 Skin			100	360 Skin					C 1* *30-min See Pocket Guide App. A	C 3.6*	20	73 Skin; C		I (2)					EPA-L IARC-2B MAK-4 NIOSH-Ca NTP-R TLV-A3
Dioxathion 78-34-2	0.1 IFV Skin; BEI_A								0.2 Skin												TLV-A4
1,3-Dioxolane 646-06-0	20	61											100	310 Skin; B		II (2)					

SUBSTANCE / CAS#	ACGIH® TLVs® TWA ppm	ACGIH® TLVs® TWA mg/m³	ACGIH® TLVs® STEL/CEIL(C) ppm	ACGIH® TLVs® STEL/CEIL(C) mg/m³	OSHA PELs TWA ppm	OSHA PELs TWA mg/m³	OSHA PELs STEL/CEIL(C) ppm	OSHA PELs STEL/CEIL(C) mg/m³	NIOSH RELs TWA ppm	NIOSH RELs TWA mg/m³	NIOSH RELs STEL/CEIL(C) ppm	NIOSH RELs STEL/CEIL(C) mg/m³	DFG MAKs TWA ppm	DFG MAKs TWA mg/m³	DFG MAKs PEAK/CEIL(C) ppm	DFG MAKs PEAK/CEIL(C) mg/m³	AIHA WEELs TWA ppm	AIHA WEELs TWA mg/m³	AIHA WEELs STEL/CEIL(C) ppm	AIHA WEELs STEL/CEIL(C) mg/m³	CARCINOGENICITY CATEGORY
Dipentamethylene-thiuram disulfide 94-37-1														Sh							
Diphenylamine 122-39-4		10								10				5 I Skin; C		II (2)					MAK-3B TLV-A4
2,4′-Diphenyldiamine 492-17-1																					IARC-3
N,N-Diphenyl-p-phenylene diamine 74-31-7														Sh							
Dipropylene glycol 25265-71-8														100 I* *sum of vapor and aerosol Skin; C		II (2)					
Dipropyl ketone 123-19-3	50	233							50	235											
Diquat 85-00-7; 2764-72-9; 6385-62-2		0.5 I 0.1 R Skin								0.5											TLV-A4
Disperse Blue 1 2475-45-8																					IARC-2B NTP-R
Disperse Blue 106/124 15141-18-1; 61951-51-7; 68516-81-4														Sh							

SUBSTANCE / CAS#	ACGIH® TLVs® TWA ppm	mg/m³	STEL/CEIL(C) ppm	mg/m³	OSHA PELs TWA ppm	mg/m³	STEL/CEIL(C) ppm	mg/m³	NIOSH RELs TWA ppm	mg/m³	STEL/CEIL(C) ppm	mg/m³	DFG MAKs TWA ppm	mg/m³	PEAK/CEIL(C) ppm	mg/m³	AIHA WEELs TWA ppm	mg/m³	STEL/CEIL(C) ppm	mg/m³	CARCINOGENICITY CATEGORY
Disperse Orange 3 730-40-5														Sh							
Disperse Red 1 2872-52-8														Sh							
Disperse Red 17 3179-89-3														Sh							
Disperse Yellow 3 2832-40-8														Sh							IARC-3
Disulfiram 97-77-8	2								2* *precautions should be taken to avoid concurrent exposure to Ethylene dibromide				2 I Sh; D		II (8)						IARC-3 TLV-A4
Disulfoton 298-04-4	0.05 **IFV** Skin; BEI$_A$								0.1 Skin												TLV-A4
1,4-Dithiane 505-29-3																					EPA-D
2,2′-Dithiobis(N-methyl-benzamide) 2527-58-4														Sh							
Dithranol 1143-38-0																					IARC-3

SUBSTANCE	ACGIH® TLVs®				OSHA PELs				NIOSH RELs				DFG MAKs				AIHA WEELs				CARCINOGENICITY CATEGORY
	TWA		STEL/CEIL(C)		TWA		STEL/CEIL(C)		TWA		STEL/CEIL(C)		TWA		PEAK/CEIL(C)		TWA		STEL/CEIL(C)		
CAS#	ppm	mg/m³	ppm	mg/m³	ppm	mg/m³	ppm	mg/m³	ppm	mg/m³	ppm	mg/m³	ppm	mg/m³	ppm	mg/m³	ppm	mg/m³	ppm	mg/m³	
Diuron		10								10											TLV-A4
330-54-1																					
Divinyl benzene	10	53							10	50											
1321-74-0																					
Dodecyl mercaptan	0.1	0.8									C 0.5*	C 4.1*									
112-55-0		(SEN) NIC-DSEN									*15-min										
Dowtherm® Q																	1				
612-00-0; 68987-42-8																					
Doxefazepam																					IARC-3
40762-15-0																					
Doxylamine succinate																					IARC-3
562-10-7																					
Droloxifene																					IARC-3
82413-20-5																					
Dulcin																					IARC-3
150-69-6																					
Dust, general threshold limit value														4 I							

SUBSTANCE CAS#	ACGIH® TLVs® TWA ppm	ACGIH® TLVs® TWA mg/m³	ACGIH® TLVs® STEL/CEIL(C) ppm	ACGIH® TLVs® STEL/CEIL(C) mg/m³	OSHA PELs TWA ppm	OSHA PELs TWA mg/m³	OSHA PELs STEL/CEIL(C) ppm	OSHA PELs STEL/CEIL(C) mg/m³	NIOSH RELs TWA ppm	NIOSH RELs TWA mg/m³	NIOSH RELs STEL/CEIL(C) ppm	NIOSH RELs STEL/CEIL(C) mg/m³	DFG MAKs TWA ppm	DFG MAKs TWA mg/m³	DFG MAKs PEAK/CEIL(C) ppm	DFG MAKs PEAK/CEIL(C) mg/m³	AIHA WEELs TWA ppm	AIHA WEELs TWA mg/m³	AIHA WEELs STEL/CEIL(C) ppm	AIHA WEELs STEL/CEIL(C) mg/m³	CARCINOGENICITY CATEGORY
Dust, general threshold limit value, biopersistent granular dusts, excluding ultrafine particles														0.3 R	II (8)						MAK-4
													for dusts with a density of 1 g/cm³ C							
Emery 1302-74-5	TLV® withdrawn; *see* Aluminum, metal and insoluble compounds				15*; 5** *Total dust **Respirable fraction									4 I 1.5 R D							
Endosulfan 115-29-7	0.006* *IFV Skin	0.1*							0.1 Skin												TLV-A4
Endrin 72-20-8	Skin	0.1			Skin	0.1			Skin	0.1			Skin; C	0.05 I	II (8)						EPA-D IARC-3 TLV-A4
Enflurane 13838-16-9	75	566			*60-min; for exposure to waste anesthetic gases				C 2*		C 15.1*		20	150 C	II (8)						IARC-3 TLV-A4
Engine exhaust																					IARC-1*; 2B** *diesel **gasoline
Eosin 15086-94-9																					IARC-3
Epichlorohydrin (1-Chloro-2,3-epoxypropane) 106-89-8	0.5 Skin	1.9			5 Skin	19			*See* Pocket Guide App. A				Skin; Sh; 3B								EPA-B2 NTP-R IARC-2A TLV-A3 MAK-2 NIOSH-Ca

SUBSTANCE / CAS#	ACGIH® TLVs® TWA ppm	ACGIH® TLVs® TWA mg/m³	ACGIH® TLVs® STEL/CEIL(C) ppm	ACGIH® TLVs® STEL/CEIL(C) mg/m³	OSHA PELs TWA ppm	OSHA PELs TWA mg/m³	OSHA PELs STEL/CEIL(C) ppm	OSHA PELs STEL/CEIL(C) mg/m³	NIOSH RELs TWA ppm	NIOSH RELs TWA mg/m³	NIOSH RELs STEL/CEIL(C) ppm	NIOSH RELs STEL/CEIL(C) mg/m³	DFG MAKs TWA ppm	DFG MAKs TWA mg/m³	DFG MAKs PEAK/CEIL(C) ppm	DFG MAKs PEAK/CEIL(C) mg/m³	AIHA WEELs TWA ppm	AIHA WEELs TWA mg/m³	AIHA WEELs STEL/CEIL(C) ppm	AIHA WEELs STEL/CEIL(C) mg/m³	CARCINOGENICITY CATEGORY
EPN (O-Ethyl O-[4-nitro-phenyl]phenylthiophos-phonate) 2104-64-5	0.1 **I** Skin; BEI_A				0.5 Skin				0.5 Skin				0.5 **I** Skin		II (2)						TLV-A4
1,2-Epoxybutane (1,2-Butylene oxide) 106-88-7														Skin				2			IARC-2B MAK-2
bis(2,3-Epoxycyclo-pentyl)ether 2386-90-5																					IARC-3
3,4-Epoxy-6-methyl-cyclohexylmethyl-3,4-epoxy-6-methyl-cyclohexane carbox-ylate 141-37-7																					IARC-3
9,10-Epoxystearic acid, cis-isomer 2443-39-2																					IARC-3
Erionite, fibrous dust 12510-42-8; 66733-21-9																					IARC-1* MAK-1 NTP-K* *CAS: 66733-21-9
Erythromycin 114-07-8																		3			IARC-3
Estazolam 29975-16-4																					IARC-3

SUBSTANCE / CAS#	ACGIH® TLVs® TWA ppm	mg/m³	STEL/CEIL(C) ppm	mg/m³	OSHA PELs TWA ppm	mg/m³	STEL/CEIL(C) ppm	mg/m³	NIOSH RELs TWA ppm	mg/m³	STEL/CEIL(C) ppm	mg/m³	DFG MAKs TWA ppm	mg/m³	PEAK/CEIL(C) ppm	mg/m³	AIHA WEELs TWA ppm	mg/m³	STEL/CEIL(C) ppm	mg/m³	CARCINOGENICITY CATEGORY
Estradiol mustard 22966-79-6																					IARC-3
Ethane 74-84-0	Refer to Appendix F: Minimal Oxygen Content																				
Ethanol (Ethyl alcohol) 64-17-5			1000	1880	1000	1900			1000	1900			500	960	II (2) C; 5						MAK-5 TLV-A3
Ethanolamine (2-Aminoethanol) 141-43-5	3	7.5	6	15	3	6			3	8	6	15	2	5.1	I (2) Sh; C						
Ethidium bromide 1239-45-8														3B							MAK-3B
Ethion 563-12-2	0.05 **IFV** Skin; BEI_A								0.4 Skin												TLV-A4
Ethionamide 536-33-4																					IARC-3
2-Ethoxyethanol (EGEE; Cellosolve) 110-80-5	5	18			200	740			0.5	1.8			2*	7.5	II (8)						
	Skin; BEI				Skin				Skin				*sum of the concentrations of EGEE and its acetate in air Skin; B								
2-(2-Ethoxyethoxy)-ethanol (Diethylene glycol-monoethyl ether) 111-90-0													50 **I** C		I (2)		25				

SUBSTANCE / CAS#	ACGIH® TLVs® TWA ppm	ACGIH® TLVs® TWA mg/m³	ACGIH® TLVs® STEL/CEIL(C) ppm	ACGIH® TLVs® STEL/CEIL(C) mg/m³	OSHA PELs TWA ppm	OSHA PELs TWA mg/m³	OSHA PELs STEL/CEIL(C) ppm	OSHA PELs STEL/CEIL(C) mg/m³	NIOSH RELs TWA ppm	NIOSH RELs TWA mg/m³	NIOSH RELs STEL/CEIL(C) ppm	NIOSH RELs STEL/CEIL(C) mg/m³	DFG MAKs TWA ppm	DFG MAKs TWA mg/m³	DFG MAKs PEAK/CEIL(C) ppm	DFG MAKs PEAK/CEIL(C) mg/m³	AIHA WEELs TWA ppm	AIHA WEELs TWA mg/m³	AIHA WEELs STEL/CEIL(C) ppm	AIHA WEELs STEL/CEIL(C) mg/m³	CARCINOGENICITY CATEGORY
2-Ethoxyethyl acetate (EGEEA; Cellosolve acetate) 111-15-9	5	27		Skin; BEI	100	540		Skin	0.5	2.7		Skin	2*	11	II (8) *sum of the concentrations of EGEE and its acetate in air Skin; B						
1-Ethoxy-2-propanol 1569-02-4													50*	220	II (2) *sum of the concentrations of CAS: 1569-02-4 and 54839-24-6 in air Skin; C						
1-Ethoxy-2-propyl acetate 54839-24-6													50*	300	II (2) *sum of the concentrations of CAS: 1569-02-4 and 54839-24-6 in air C						
Ethyl acetate 141-78-6	400	1440			400	1400			400	1400			400	1500	I (2) C						
Ethyl acrylate (Acrylic acid, ethyl ester) 140-88-5	5	20	15	61	25	100		Skin				*See* Pocket Guide App. A	5	21	I (2) Sh; C						IARC-2B NIOSH-Ca TLV-A4
Ethylamine 75-04-7	5	9	15	28 Skin	10	18			10	18			5	9.4	I (2) C 10 19 D						
Ethyl amyl ketone (5-Methyl-3-heptanone) 541-85-5	10	52			25	130			25	130			10	53	I (2) D						
Ethyl benzene 100-41-4	20	87	125	543 BEI	100	435			100	435	125	545	20	88	II (2) Skin; C						EPA-D IARC-2B MAK-4 TLV-A3
Ethyl bromide (Bromoethane) 74-96-4	5	22		Skin	200	890									Skin							IARC-3 MAK-2 TLV-A3

SUBSTANCE	ACGIH® TLVs®				OSHA PELs				NIOSH RELs				DFG MAKs				AIHA WEELs				CARCINOGENICITY CATEGORY
	TWA		STEL/CEIL(C)		TWA		STEL/CEIL(C)		TWA		STEL/CEIL(C)		TWA		PEAK/CEIL(C)		TWA		STEL/CEIL(C)		
CAS#	ppm	mg/m³	ppm	mg/m³	ppm	mg/m³	ppm	mg/m³	ppm	mg/m³	ppm	mg/m³	ppm	mg/m³	ppm	mg/m³	ppm	mg/m³	ppm	mg/m³	
Ethyl tert-butyl ether 637-92-3	25	105																			TLV-A4
Ethyl butyl ketone (3-Heptanone) 106-35-4	50	234	75	350	50	230			50	230			10	47	I (2) D						
Ethyl chloride (Chloroethane) 75-00-3	100	264		Skin	1000	2600			handle with caution *See* Pocket Guide App. C					Skin							IARC-3 MAK-3B TLV-A3
Ethyl chloroformate (Chloroformic acid ethyl ester) 541-41-3																					MAK-3B
Ethyl cyanoacrylate (Ethyl 2-cyanoacrylate) 7085-85-0	0.2	1																			
5-Ethyl-3,7-dioxa-1-aza- bicyclo[3.3.0]octane 7747-35-5														Sh							
Ethylene 74-85-1	200	230																			IARC-3 MAK-3B TLV-A4
Ethylene chlorohydrin (2-Chloroethanol) 107-07-3			C 1	C 3.3	5	16		Skin			C 1	C 3	1	3.3	II (1)						TLV-A4
				Skin								Skin			Skin; C						
Ethylenediamine (1,2-Diaminoethane) 107-15-3	10	25		Skin	10	25			10	25					Sah						EPA-D TLV-A4

SUBSTANCE / CAS#	ACGIH® TLVs® TWA ppm	TWA mg/m³	STEL/CEIL(C) ppm	STEL/CEIL(C) mg/m³	OSHA PELs TWA ppm	TWA mg/m³	STEL/CEIL(C) ppm	STEL/CEIL(C) mg/m³	NIOSH RELs TWA ppm	TWA mg/m³	STEL/CEIL(C) ppm	STEL/CEIL(C) mg/m³	DFG MAKs TWA ppm	TWA mg/m³	PEAK/CEIL(C) ppm	PEAK/CEIL(C) mg/m³	AIHA WEELs TWA ppm	TWA mg/m³	STEL/CEIL(C) ppm	STEL/CEIL(C) mg/m³	CARCINOGENICITY CATEGORY
Ethylene dibromide (1,2-Dibromoethane) 106-93-4		Skin			20		C 30; 50* *5-min peak per 8-hr shift		0.045		C 0.13* *15-min See Pocket Guide App. A			Skin							EPA-L NTP-R IARC-2A TLV-A3 MAK-2 NIOSH-Ca
Ethylene dichloride (1,2-Dichloroethane) 107-06-2	10	40			50		C 100; 200* *5-min peak in any 3 hrs		1	4	2	8		Skin							EPA-B2 NIOSH-Ca IARC-2B NTP-R MAK-2 TLV-A4 See Pocket Guide Apps. A and C
Ethylene glycol 107-21-1		H	C 100										10	26	I (2) Skin; C						TLV-A4
Ethylene glycol dimeth-acrylate 97-90-5														Sh							
Ethylene glycol dinitrate (EGDN) 628-96-6	0.05	0.31					C 0.2	C 1				0.1	0.05	0.32	II (1)						
		Skin				Skin				Skin				Skin							
Ethylene glycol methacrylate (2-Hydroxy-ethyl methacrylate) 868-77-9														Sh							
Ethylene oxide (EtO) 75-21-8	1	1.8			1 See 29 CFR 1910.1047(c)		5		< 0.1	0.18	C 5* *10-min/day See Pocket Guide App. A	C 9*		Skin; 2							IARC-1 OSHA-Ca MAK-2 TLV-A2 NIOSH-Ca NTP-K
Ethylene sulfide 420-12-2																					IARC-3
Ethylene thiourea 96-45-7									use encapsulated form See Pocket Guide App. A												IARC-3 MAK-3B NIOSH-Ca NTP-R

SUBSTANCE CAS#	ACGIH® TLVs® TWA ppm	mg/m³	STEL/CEIL(C) ppm	mg/m³	OSHA PELs TWA ppm	mg/m³	STEL/CEIL(C) ppm	mg/m³	NIOSH RELs TWA ppm	mg/m³	STEL/CEIL(C) ppm	mg/m³	DFG MAKs TWA ppm	mg/m³	PEAK/CEIL(C) ppm	mg/m³	AIHA WEELs TWA ppm	mg/m³	STEL/CEIL(C) ppm	mg/m³	CARCINOGENICITY CATEGORY
Ethyleneimine 151-56-4	0.05	0.09	0.1	0.18 Skin	See 29 CFR 1910.1003				See Pocket Guide App. A				400	1200 Skin; 2							IARC-2B TLV-A3 MAK-2 NIOSH-Ca OSHA-Ca
Ethyl ether (Diethyl ether) 60-29-7	400	1210	500	1520	400	1200							400	1200 D	I (1)						
Ethyl-3-ethoxy-propionate 763-69-9													100	610 Skin; C	I (1)						
Ethyl formate (Formic acid, ethyl ester) 109-94-4			100	303	100	300			100	300			100	310 Skin; C	I (1)						TLV-A4
2-Ethylhexanoic acid 149-57-5	5 **IFV**																				
2-Ethylhexanol 104-76-7													10	54 C	I (1)						
2-Ethylhexyl acrylate (Acrylic acid, 2-ethylhexyl ester) 103-11-7													5	38 Sh; C	I (1)						IARC-3
Ethylidene norbornene 16219-75-3	NIC-2	NIC-10	(C 5) NIC-4	(C 25) NIC-20							C 5	C 25									
Ethyl isocyanate 109-90-0	NIC-0.02	NIC-0.06	NIC-0.06	NIC-0.17 NIC-Skin; DSEN																	

SUBSTANCE / CAS#	ACGIH® TLVs® TWA ppm	TWA mg/m³	STEL/CEIL(C) ppm	STEL/CEIL(C) mg/m³	OSHA PELs TWA ppm	TWA mg/m³	STEL/CEIL(C) ppm	STEL/CEIL(C) mg/m³	NIOSH RELs TWA ppm	TWA mg/m³	STEL/CEIL(C) ppm	STEL/CEIL(C) mg/m³	DFG MAKs TWA ppm	TWA mg/m³	PEAK/CEIL(C) ppm	PEAK/CEIL(C) mg/m³	AIHA WEELs TWA ppm	TWA mg/m³	STEL/CEIL(C) ppm	STEL/CEIL(C) mg/m³	CARCINOGENICITY CATEGORY
Ethyl mercaptan (Ethanethiol) 75-08-1	0.5	1.3					C 10	C 25			C 0.5* *15 min	C 1.3*	0.5	1.3 D	II (2)						
Ethyl methacrylate (Methacrylic acid, ethyl ester) 97-63-2														Sh							
Ethyl methanesulfonate 62-50-0																					IARC-2B NTP-R
Ethyl methyl ketoxime (2-Butanone oxime) 96-29-7														Skin; Sh			10		DSEN		MAK-2
N-Ethylmorpholine 100-74-3	5	24	Skin		20	94	Skin		5	23	Skin										
Ethyl selenac 5456-28-0																					IARC-3
Ethyl silicate (Silicic acid tetraethyl ester) 78-10-4	10	85			100	850			10	85			10	86 D	I (1)						
Ethyl telluric 20941-65-5																					IARC-3
Etoposide 33419-42-0																					IARC-1

SUBSTANCE CAS#	ACGIH® TLVs® TWA ppm	mg/m³	STEL/CEIL(C) ppm	mg/m³	OSHA PELs TWA ppm	mg/m³	STEL/CEIL(C) ppm	mg/m³	NIOSH RELs TWA ppm	mg/m³	STEL/CEIL(C) ppm	mg/m³	DFG MAKs TWA ppm	mg/m³	PEAK/CEIL(C) ppm	mg/m³	AIHA WEELs TWA ppm	mg/m³	STEL/CEIL(C) ppm	mg/m³	CARCINOGENICITY CATEGORY
Eugenol 97-53-0														Sh							IARC-3
Evans Blue 314-13-6																					IARC-3
Farnesol 4602-84-0														Sh							
Fast Green FCF 2353-45-9																					IARC-3
Fenamiphos 22224-92-6	0.05 IFV Skin; BEI_A								0.1 Skin												TLV-A4
Fensulfothion 115-90-2	0.01 IFV Skin; BEI_A								0.1												TLV-A4
Fenthion 55-38-9	0.05 IFV Skin; BEI_A												0.2 I		II (2) Skin						TLV-A4
Fenvalerate 51630-58-1																					IARC-3
Ferbam 14484-64-1	5 I					15* *Total dust				10											IARC-3 TLV-A4

SUBSTANCE CAS#	ACGIH® TLVs® TWA ppm	ACGIH® TLVs® TWA mg/m³	ACGIH® TLVs® STEL/CEIL(C) ppm	ACGIH® TLVs® STEL/CEIL(C) mg/m³	OSHA PELs TWA ppm	OSHA PELs TWA mg/m³	OSHA PELs STEL/CEIL(C) ppm	OSHA PELs STEL/CEIL(C) mg/m³	NIOSH RELs TWA ppm	NIOSH RELs TWA mg/m³	NIOSH RELs STEL/CEIL(C) ppm	NIOSH RELs STEL/CEIL(C) mg/m³	DFG MAKs TWA ppm	DFG MAKs TWA mg/m³	DFG MAKs PEAK/CEIL(C) ppm	DFG MAKs PEAK/CEIL(C) mg/m³	AIHA WEELs TWA ppm	AIHA WEELs TWA mg/m³	AIHA WEELs STEL/CEIL(C) ppm	AIHA WEELs STEL/CEIL(C) mg/m³	CARCINOGENICITY CATEGORY
Ferrovanadium dust 12604-58-9		1		3		1				1		3									
Flour dust		0.5 I												Cereal (rye, wheat) flour dusts							
		(SEN) NIC-RSEN												Sa							
Fluometuron 2164-17-2																					IARC-3
Fluoranthene 206-44-0																					EPA-D IARC-3
Fluorene 86-73-7																					EPA-D IARC-3
Fluorides, as F		2.5				2.5				2.5			1 I		II (4)						IARC-3* TLV-A4 *inorganic, used in drinking water
		BEI												Skin; C							
Fluorine 7782-41-4	1	1.6	2	3.1	0.1	0.2			0.1	0.2											
5-Fluorouracil 51-21-8																					IARC-3
Fluroxene 406-90-6											C 2*	C 10.3*									
									*60-min; for exposure to waste anesthetic gases												

SUBSTANCE CAS#	ACGIH® TLVs® TWA ppm	mg/m³	STEL/CEIL(C) ppm	mg/m³	OSHA PELs TWA ppm	mg/m³	STEL/CEIL(C) ppm	mg/m³	NIOSH RELs TWA ppm	mg/m³	STEL/CEIL(C) ppm	mg/m³	DFG MAKs TWA ppm	mg/m³	PEAK/CEIL(C) ppm	mg/m³	AIHA WEELs TWA ppm	mg/m³	STEL/CEIL(C) ppm	mg/m³	CARCINOGENICITY CATEGORY
Folpet 133-07-3																					EPA-B2
Fomesafen 72178-02-0																					EPA-C
Fonofos 944-22-9	0.1 **IFV** Skin; BEI_A								0.1 Skin												TLV-A4
Formaldehyde 50-00-0			C 0.3 SEN	C 0.37	0.75 See 29 CFR 1910.1048(c)		2		0.016 See Pocket Guide App. A		C 0.1* *15-min		0.3 Sh; C; 5	0.37	I (2) C 1	C 1.2					EPA-B1 NTP-K IARC-1 OSHA-Ca MAK-4 TLV-A2 NIOSH-Ca
Formaldehyde condensation products with p-tert-butylphenol (low-molecular)													Sh								
Formaldehyde condensation products with phenol (low-molecular)													Sh								
Formamide 75-12-7	10 Skin	18							10 Skin	15			Skin								
Formic acid 64-18-6	5	9.4	10	19	5	9			5	9			5 C	9.5	I (2)						
Fosetyl-al 39148-24-8																					EPA-C

SUBSTANCE / CAS#	ACGIH TLVs TWA ppm	mg/m³	STEL/CEIL(C) ppm	mg/m³	OSHA PELs TWA ppm	mg/m³	STEL/CEIL(C) ppm	mg/m³	NIOSH RELs TWA ppm	mg/m³	STEL/CEIL(C) ppm	mg/m³	DFG MAKs TWA ppm	mg/m³	PEAK/CEIL(C) ppm	mg/m³	AIHA WEELs TWA ppm	mg/m³	STEL/CEIL(C) ppm	mg/m³	CARCINOGENICITY CATEGORY
Fuel oils, distillate (light)																					IARC-3
Fumonisin B₁ 116355-83-0																					IARC-2B
Furan 110-00-9														Skin				(W)			IARC-2B MAK-2 NTP-R
Furazolidone 67-45-8																					IARC-3
Furfural 98-01-1	2	7.9 Skin; BEI			5	20 Skin								Skin							IARC-3 MAK-3B TLV-A3
Furfuryl alcohol 98-00-0	10	40 Skin	15	60	50	200			10	40 Skin	15	60		Skin							MAK-3B
Furmecyclox 60568-05-0																					EPA-B2
Furosemide (Frusemide) 54-31-9																					IARC-3
Furothiazole 531-82-8																					IARC-2B

SUBSTANCE / CAS#	ACGIH® TLVs® TWA ppm	mg/m³	STEL/CEIL(C) ppm	mg/m³	OSHA PELs TWA ppm	mg/m³	STEL/CEIL(C) ppm	mg/m³	NIOSH RELs TWA ppm	mg/m³	STEL/CEIL(C) ppm	mg/m³	DFG MAKs TWA ppm	mg/m³	PEAK/CEIL(C) ppm	mg/m³	AIHA WEELs TWA ppm	mg/m³	STEL/CEIL(C) ppm	mg/m³	CARCINOGENICITY CATEGORY
Furylfuramide 3688-53-7																					IARC-2B
Gallium arsenide 1303-00-0	0.0003 R										C 0.002* as As *15-min See Pocket Guide App. A										IARC-1* NIOSH-Ca TLV-A3 *as As
Gasoline 86290-81-5; 8006-61-9	300	890	500	1480 bulk handling					See Pocket Guide App. A												IARC-2B NIOSH-Ca TLV-A3
Gemfibrozil 25812-30-0																					IARC-3
Geraniol 106-24-1														Sh							
Germanium tetra-hydride 7782-65-2	0.2	0.63							0.2	0.6											
Glutaraldehyde 111-30-8			C 0.05 activated or inactivated SEN	C 0.2							C 0.2 See Pocket Guide App. C	C 0.8	0.05	0.21 Sah; C	I (2) C 0.2	C 0.83					MAK-4 TLV-A4
Glycerin 56-81-5		Mist TLV® withdrawn due to insufficient data relevant to human occupational exposure			15*; 5** Mist *Total dust **Respirable fraction								50 I	C	I (2)						
Glyceryl monothio-glycolate 30618-84-9														Sh							

SUBSTANCE / CAS#	ACGIH® TLVs® TWA ppm	TWA mg/m³	STEL/CEIL(C) ppm	STEL/CEIL(C) mg/m³	OSHA PELs TWA ppm	TWA mg/m³	STEL/CEIL(C) ppm	STEL/CEIL(C) mg/m³	NIOSH RELs TWA ppm	TWA mg/m³	STEL/CEIL(C) ppm	STEL/CEIL(C) mg/m³	DFG MAKs TWA ppm	TWA mg/m³	PEAK/CEIL(C) ppm	PEAK/CEIL(C) mg/m³	AIHA WEELs TWA ppm	TWA mg/m³	STEL/CEIL(C) ppm	STEL/CEIL(C) mg/m³	CARCINOGENICITY CATEGORY
Glycidaldehyde 765-34-4																					EPA-B2 IARC-2B
Glycidol (2,3-Epoxy-1-propanol) 556-52-5	2	6.1			50	150			25	75						Skin					IARC-2A MAK-2 NTP-R TLV-A3
Glycidyl methacrylate 106-91-2																		0.5		Skin; DSEN	
Glycidyl oleate 5431-33-4																					IARC-3
Glycidyl stearate 7460-84-6																					IARC-3
Glycidyl trimethyl ammonium chloride 3033-77-0																Skin; Sh					MAK-2
Glycolonitrile 107-16-4											C 2* *15-min	C 5*									
Glyoxal 107-22-2		0.1 IFV (SEN) NIC-DSEN														Skin; Sh		0.1 DSEN; (H)			MAK-3B TLV-A4
Glyphosate 1071-83-6																					EPA-D

SUBSTANCE / CAS#	ACGIH® TLVs® TWA ppm	mg/m³	STEL/CEIL(C) ppm	mg/m³	OSHA PELs TWA ppm	mg/m³	STEL/CEIL(C) ppm	mg/m³	NIOSH RELs TWA ppm	mg/m³	STEL/CEIL(C) ppm	mg/m³	DFG MAKs TWA ppm	mg/m³	PEAK/CEIL(C) ppm	mg/m³	AIHA WEELs TWA ppm	mg/m³	STEL/CEIL(C) ppm	mg/m³	CARCINOGENICITY CATEGORY
Gold [7440-57-5] and inorganic compounds														soluble compounds only Sh							
Grain dust (oat; wheat; barley)	4				10				4												
Graphite, natural 7782-42-5		2 R all forms except Graphite fibers			15 mppcf* *based on impinger samples counted by light field techniques				2.5* *Respirable dust					1.5 R 4 I C							
Graphite, synthetic		2 R all forms except Graphite fibers			15*; 5** *Total dust **Respirable fraction																
Griseofulvin 126-07-8																					IARC-2B
Guinea Green B 4680-78-8																					IARC-3
Gyromitrin 16568-02-8																					IARC-3
Hafnium [7440-58-6] and compounds, as Hf		0.5				0.5				0.5											
Halloysite, fibrous dust 12298-43-0																					MAK-3B

SUBSTANCE / CAS#	ACGIH® TLVs® TWA ppm	ACGIH® TLVs® TWA mg/m³	ACGIH® TLVs® STEL/CEIL(C) ppm	ACGIH® TLVs® STEL/CEIL(C) mg/m³	OSHA PELs TWA ppm	OSHA PELs TWA mg/m³	OSHA PELs STEL/CEIL(C) ppm	OSHA PELs STEL/CEIL(C) mg/m³	NIOSH RELs TWA ppm	NIOSH RELs TWA mg/m³	NIOSH RELs STEL/CEIL(C) ppm	NIOSH RELs STEL/CEIL(C) mg/m³	DFG MAKs TWA ppm	DFG MAKs TWA mg/m³	DFG MAKs PEAK/CEIL(C) ppm	DFG MAKs PEAK/CEIL(C) mg/m³	AIHA WEELs TWA ppm	AIHA WEELs TWA mg/m³	AIHA WEELs STEL/CEIL(C) ppm	AIHA WEELs STEL/CEIL(C) mg/m³	CARCINOGENICITY CATEGORY
Halothane 151-67-7	50	404									C 2*	C 16.2*	5	41	II (8)						IARC-3 TLV-A4
									*60-min; for exposure to waste anesthetic gases				B								
Hard metal containing tungsten carbide and cobalt													Inhalable fraction Skin; Sah; 3A								MAK-1
HC Blue No. 1 2784-94-3																					IARC-2B
HC Blue No. 2 33229-34-4																					IARC-3
HC Red No. 3 2871-01-4																					IARC-3
HC Yellow No. 4 59820-43-8																					IARC-3
Helium 7440-59-7	NIC-withdraw TLV®; refer to Appendix F: Minimal Oxygen Content (Simple asphyxiant (D))																				
Hematite 1317-60-8																					IARC-3; 1* *mining underground
Heptachlor 76-44-8	0.05 Skin				0.5 Skin				0.5 Skin See Pocket Guide App. A				0.05 I Skin; D		II (8)						EPA-B2 TLV-A3 IARC-2B MAK-4 NIOSH-Ca

SUBSTANCE CAS#	ACGIH® TLVs® TWA ppm	mg/m³	STEL/CEIL(C) ppm	mg/m³	OSHA PELs TWA ppm	mg/m³	STEL/CEIL(C) ppm	mg/m³	NIOSH RELs TWA ppm	mg/m³	STEL/CEIL(C) ppm	mg/m³	DFG MAKs TWA ppm	mg/m³	PEAK/CEIL(C) ppm	mg/m³	AIHA WEELs TWA ppm	mg/m³	STEL/CEIL(C) ppm	mg/m³	CARCINOGENICITY CATEGORY
Heptachlor epoxide 1024-57-3		0.05		Skin																	EPA-B2 IARC-2B TLV-A3
Heptane, all isomers 108-08-7; 142-82-5; 565-59-3; 589-34-4; 590-35-2; 591-76-4	400	1640	500	2050	500	2000		CAS: 142-82-5 only	85	350	C 440* *15-min CAS: 142-82-5 only	C 1800*	500	2100 CAS: 142-82-5 only	I (1) D						EPA-D* *CAS: 142-82-5 only
n-Heptyl mercaptan (1-Heptanethiol) 1639-09-4											C 0.5* *15-min	C 2.7*									
Hexabromodiphenyl ether 36483-60-0																					EPA-D
2,2′,4,4′,5,5′-Hexabromodiphenyl ether (BDE-153) 68631-49-2																					EPA-I
Hexachlorobenzene (HCB) 118-74-1		0.002		Skin										Skin; D							EPA-B2 TLV-A3 IARC-2B MAK-4 NTP-R
Hexachlorobutadiene 87-68-3	0.02	0.21		Skin					0.02	0.24 Skin See Pocket Guide App. A				Skin							EPA-C TLV-A3 IARC-3 MAK-3B NIOSH-Ca
1,2,3,4,5,6-Hexachloro-cyclohexane, mixture of α-HCH [319-84-6] and β-HCH [319-85-7] isomers														0.1* I *(concentration α-HCH ÷ 5) + concentration β-HCH Skin; D	II (8)						EPA-B2*; C** MAK-4 *319-84-6 **319-85-7

SUBSTANCE / CAS#	ACGIH® TLVs® TWA ppm	ACGIH® TLVs® TWA mg/m³	ACGIH® TLVs® STEL/CEIL(C) ppm	ACGIH® TLVs® STEL/CEIL(C) mg/m³	OSHA PELs TWA ppm	OSHA PELs TWA mg/m³	OSHA PELs STEL/CEIL(C) ppm	OSHA PELs STEL/CEIL(C) mg/m³	NIOSH RELs TWA ppm	NIOSH RELs TWA mg/m³	NIOSH RELs STEL/CEIL(C) ppm	NIOSH RELs STEL/CEIL(C) mg/m³	DFG MAKs TWA ppm	DFG MAKs TWA mg/m³	DFG MAKs PEAK/CEIL(C) ppm	DFG MAKs PEAK/CEIL(C) mg/m³	AIHA WEELs TWA ppm	AIHA WEELs TWA mg/m³	AIHA WEELs STEL/CEIL(C) ppm	AIHA WEELs STEL/CEIL(C) mg/m³	CARCINOGENICITY CATEGORY
Hexachlorocyclohex-ane technical (t-HCH) 608-73-1																					EPA-B2
α-Hexachlorocyclo-hexane 319-84-6														0.5 I		II (8)					MAK-4
														Skin; D							
Δ-Hexachlorocyclo-hexane 319-86-8																					EPA-D
ε-Hexachlorocyclo-hexane 6108-10-7																					EPA-D
Hexachlorocyclo-pentadiene 77-47-4	0.01	0.11							0.01	0.1											EPA-NL; E TLV-A4
														Skin							
Hexachlorodibenzo-p-dioxin, mixture (HxCDD) 19408-74-3; 57653-85-7																					EPA-B2
Hexachloroethane 67-72-1	1	9.7			1	10			1	10			1	9.8		II (2)					EPA-L TLV-A3 IARC-2B NIOSH-Ca NTP-R
		Skin				Skin			Skin *See* Pocket Guide Apps. A and C												
Hexachloronaphthalene 1335-87-1		0.2				0.2				0.2											
		Skin				Skin				Skin				Skin							
Hexachlorophene 70-30-4																					IARC-3

SUBSTANCE CAS#	ACGIH® TLVs® TWA ppm	ACGIH® TLVs® TWA mg/m³	ACGIH® TLVs® STEL/CEIL(C) ppm	ACGIH® TLVs® STEL/CEIL(C) mg/m³	OSHA PELs TWA ppm	OSHA PELs TWA mg/m³	OSHA PELs STEL/CEIL(C) ppm	OSHA PELs STEL/CEIL(C) mg/m³	NIOSH RELs TWA ppm	NIOSH RELs TWA mg/m³	NIOSH RELs STEL/CEIL(C) ppm	NIOSH RELs STEL/CEIL(C) mg/m³	DFG MAKs TWA ppm	DFG MAKs TWA mg/m³	DFG MAKs PEAK/CEIL(C) ppm	DFG MAKs PEAK/CEIL(C) mg/m³	AIHA WEELs TWA ppm	AIHA WEELs TWA mg/m³	AIHA WEELs STEL/CEIL(C) ppm	AIHA WEELs STEL/CEIL(C) mg/m³	CARCINOGENICITY CATEGORY
2,4-Hexadienal 142-83-6																					IARC-2B
1,4-Hexadiene 592-45-0																	10	34			
Hexafluoroacetone 684-16-2	0.1	0.68 Skin							0.1	0.7 Skin											
1,1,1,3,3,3-Hexa-fluoropropane 690-39-1																	1000				
Hexafluoropropylene 116-15-4	0.1	0.6																			
Hexahydrophthalic anhy-dride, all isomers 85-42-7; 13149-00-3; 14166-21-3		(SEN) NIC-DSEN; RSEN	C 0.005 **IFV**										CAS: 85-42-7 Sa								
Hexamethylene bis(3-[3,5-di-*tert*-butyl-4-hy-droxyphenyl]propio-nate) 35074-77-2													10 **I** C	**II (2)**							
1,6-Hexamethylene diisocyanate 822-06-0	0.005	0.034							0.005	0.035 *10-min	C 0.02*	C 0.14*	0.005 Sah; D	0.035	**I (1)** C 0.01	C 0.07					

SUBSTANCE / CAS#	ACGIH® TLVs® TWA ppm	mg/m³	STEL/CEIL(C) ppm	mg/m³	OSHA PELs TWA ppm	mg/m³	STEL/CEIL(C) ppm	mg/m³	NIOSH RELs TWA ppm	mg/m³	STEL/CEIL(C) ppm	mg/m³	DFG MAKs TWA ppm	mg/m³	PEAK/CEIL(C) ppm	mg/m³	AIHA WEELs TWA ppm	mg/m³	STEL/CEIL(C) ppm	mg/m³	CARCINOGENICITY CATEGORY
Hexamethylene glycol 629-11-8																		10			
Hexamethylene-tetramine 100-97-0														Sh							
Hexamethyl phos-phoramide 680-31-9		Skin							See Pocket Guide App. A					Skin; 2							IARC-2B TLV-A3 MAK-2 NIOSH-Ca NTP-R
n-Hexane (Hexane) 110-54-3	50	176 Skin; BEI			500	1800			50	180			50	180 C	II (8)						EPA-II
Hexane, isomers, other than n-Hexane 75-83-2; 79-29-8; 96-14-0; 107-83-5	500	1760	1000	3500					100	350	C 510*	C 1800* *15-min	500	1800 D	II (2) including CAS: 96-37-7						
1,6-Hexanediamine 124-09-4	0.5	2.3																1			
1,6-Hexanediol diacrylate 13048-33-4														Sh				1		DSEN	
1-Hexene 592-41-6	50	172																			
sec-Hexyl acetate 108-84-9	50	295			50	300			50	300											

SUBSTANCE / CAS#	ACGIH® TLVs® TWA ppm	mg/m³	STEL/CEIL(C) ppm	mg/m³	OSHA PELs TWA ppm	mg/m³	STEL/CEIL(C) ppm	mg/m³	NIOSH RELs TWA ppm	mg/m³	STEL/CEIL(C) ppm	mg/m³	DFG MAKs TWA ppm	mg/m³	PEAK/CEIL(C) ppm	mg/m³	AIHA WEELs TWA ppm	mg/m³	STEL/CEIL(C) ppm	mg/m³	CARCINOGENICITY CATEGORY
n-Hexyl alcohol 111-27-3																	40	eye irritation			
Hexylene glycol 107-41-5			C 25	C 121							C 25	C 125	10	49	I (2)						D
n-Hexyl mercaptan (n-Hexanethiol) 111-31-9											C 0.5*	C 2.7* *15-min									
HFE-7100 163702-07-6; 163702-08-7																	750				
Hycanthone mesylate 23255-93-8																					IARC-3
Hydralazine 86-54-4																					IARC-3
Hydrazine 302-01-2	0.01	0.013			1	1.3					C 0.03*	C 0.04* *120-min									EPA-B2 NTP-R IARC-2B TLV-A3 MAK-2 NIOSH-Ca
		Skin				Skin			See Pocket Guide App. A					Skin; Sh							
Hydrazine hydrate and hydrazine salts 7803-57-8														Sh							
Hydrazine sulfate 10034-93-2																					NTP-R

SUBSTANCE CAS#	ACGIH® TLVs® TWA ppm	ACGIH® TLVs® TWA mg/m³	ACGIH® TLVs® STEL/CEIL(C) ppm	ACGIH® TLVs® STEL/CEIL(C) mg/m³	OSHA PELs TWA ppm	OSHA PELs TWA mg/m³	OSHA PELs STEL/CEIL(C) ppm	OSHA PELs STEL/CEIL(C) mg/m³	NIOSH RELs TWA ppm	NIOSH RELs TWA mg/m³	NIOSH RELs STEL/CEIL(C) ppm	NIOSH RELs STEL/CEIL(C) mg/m³	DFG MAKs TWA ppm	DFG MAKs TWA mg/m³	DFG MAKs PEAK/CEIL(C) ppm	DFG MAKs PEAK/CEIL(C) mg/m³	AIHA WEELs TWA ppm	AIHA WEELs TWA mg/m³	AIHA WEELs STEL/CEIL(C) ppm	AIHA WEELs STEL/CEIL(C) mg/m³	CARCINOGENICITY CATEGORY
Hydrazobenzene (1,2-Diphenylhydrazine) 122-66-7																					EPA-B2 MAK-2 NTP-R
Hydrazoic acid 7782-79-8													0.1	0.18	I (2)						
Hydrogen 1333-74-0	NIC-withdraw TLV®; refer to Appendix F: Minimal Oxygen Content (Simple asphyxiant (D))																				
Hydrogenated ter-phenyls 61788-32-7	0.5	4.9 Nonirradiated							0.5	5											
Hydrogen bromide 10035-10-6			C 2	C 6.8	3	10					C 3	C 10	2	6.7	I (1) D						
Hydrogen chloride 7647-01-0			C 2	C 2.98	−		C 5	C 7			C 5	C 7	2	3	I (2) C						IARC-3 TLV-A4
Hydrochlorothiazide 58-93-5																					IARC-3
Hydrogen cyanide 74-90-8			C 4.7* *as CN. Skin	C 5** **Cyanide salts, as CN	10	11 Skin					4.7 Skin	5	1.9	2.1 Skin; C	II (2)						EPA-II* *and Cyanide salts
Hydrogen fluoride, as F 7664-39-3	0.5	0.41 Skin; BEI	C 2	C 1.64	3				3	2.5	C 6* *15-min	C 5*	1	0.83 C	I (2)						

SUBSTANCE / CAS#	ACGIH® TLVs® TWA ppm	mg/m³	STEL/CEIL(C) ppm	mg/m³	OSHA PELs TWA ppm	mg/m³	STEL/CEIL(C) ppm	mg/m³	NIOSH RELs TWA ppm	mg/m³	STEL/CEIL(C) ppm	mg/m³	DFG MAKs TWA ppm	mg/m³	PEAK/CEIL(C) ppm	mg/m³	AIHA WEELs TWA ppm	mg/m³	STEL/CEIL(C) ppm	mg/m³	CARCINOGENICITY CATEGORY
Hydrogen peroxide 7722-84-1	1	1.4			1	1.4			1	1.4			0.5	0.71	I (1) C						IARC-3 MAK-4 TLV-A3
Hydrogen selenide 7783-07-5	0.05	0.16			0.05*	0.2* *as Se			0.05	0.2			0.006	0.02	II (8) C						MAK-3B
Hydrogen sulfide 7783-06-4	1	1.4	5	7		C 20; 50* *10-min peak; once per 8-hr shift					C 10* *10-min	C 15*	5	7.1	I (2) C						EPA-I
Hydroquinone (Dihydroxybenzene) 123-31-9		1 (SEN) NIC-DSEN				2					C 2* *15-min		Skin; Sh; 3A								IARC-3 MAK-2 TLV-A3
1-Hydroxyanthra-quinone 129-43-1																					IARC-2B
4-Hydroxyazobenzene 1689-82-3																					IARC-3
Hydroxybenzoic acid 99-96-7																		5			
Hydroxycitronellal 107-75-5													Sh								
2-Hydroxyethyl acrylate 818-61-1													Sh								

SUBSTANCE / CAS#	ACGIH® TLVs® TWA ppm	mg/m³	STEL/CEIL(C) ppm	mg/m³	OSHA PELs TWA ppm	mg/m³	STEL/CEIL(C) ppm	mg/m³	NIOSH RELs TWA ppm	mg/m³	STEL/CEIL(C) ppm	mg/m³	DFG MAKs TWA ppm	mg/m³	PEAK/CEIL(C) ppm	mg/m³	AIHA WEELs TWA ppm	mg/m³	STEL/CEIL(C) ppm	mg/m³	CARCINOGENICITY CATEGORY
N,N′,N″-tris(β-Hydroxy-ethyl)-hexahydro-1,3,5-triazine 4719-04-4														Sh							
Hydroxylamine and its salts 7803-49-8														Sh							
4-(4-Hydroxy-4-methylpentyl)-3-cyclohexene-1-carboxalde-hyde (Lyral) 31906-04-4														Sh							
Hydroxypropyl acrylate, all isomers (Acrylic acid hy-droxypropyl ester) 25584-83-2														Sh							
2-Hydroxypropyl acrylate 999-61-1	0.5	2.8							0.5	3											
	Skin; (SEN) NIC-DSEN								Skin					Sh							
2-Hydroxypropyl methacry-late (Methacrylic acid 2-hy-droxypropyl ester) 923-26-2														Sh							
8-Hydroxyquinoline 148-24-3																					IARC-3
Hydroxysenkirkine 26782-43-4																					IARC-3
Hydroxyurea 127-07-1																					IARC-3

SUBSTANCE / CAS#	ACGIH® TLVs® TWA ppm	mg/m³	STEL/CEIL(C) ppm	mg/m³	OSHA PELs TWA ppm	mg/m³	STEL/CEIL(C) ppm	mg/m³	NIOSH RELs TWA ppm	mg/m³	STEL/CEIL(C) ppm	mg/m³	DFG MAKs TWA ppm	mg/m³	PEAK/CEIL(C) ppm	mg/m³	AIHA WEELs TWA ppm	mg/m³	STEL/CEIL(C) ppm	mg/m³	CARCINOGENICITY CATEGORY
Hypochlorite salts																					IARC-3
Indene 95-13-6	5	24							10	45											
Indeno[1,2,3,cd]pyrene 193-39-5													Skin								EPA-B2 IARC-2B MAK-2 NTP-R
Indium [7440-74-6] and compounds, as In		0.1								0.1											
Indium phosphide 22398-80-7																					IARC-2A MAK-2
Iodides	0.01 IFV																				TLV-A4
Iodine 7553-56-2	0.01* *IFV	0.1*	0.1 (V)	1			C 0.1	C 1			C 0.1	C 1									TLV-A4
Iodoform 75-47-8	0.6	10							0.6	10											
3-Iodo-2-propynyl butylcarbamate 55406-53-6													0.01	0.12	I (2) Sh; C						

SUBSTANCE / CAS#	ACGIH® TLVs® TWA ppm	mg/m³	STEL/CEIL(C) ppm	mg/m³	OSHA PELs TWA ppm	mg/m³	STEL/CEIL(C) ppm	mg/m³	NIOSH RELs TWA ppm	mg/m³	STEL/CEIL(C) ppm	mg/m³	DFG MAKs TWA ppm	mg/m³	PEAK/CEIL(C) ppm	mg/m³	AIHA WEELs TWA ppm	mg/m³	STEL/CEIL(C) ppm	mg/m³	CARCINOGENICITY CATEGORY
Iron-dextran complex 9004-66-4																					IARC-2B NTP-R
Iron-dextrin complex 9004-51-7																					IARC-3
Iron oxide (FeO) 1345-25-1														with the exception of Iron oxides which are not biologically available							MAK-3B
Iron oxide (Fe₂O₃) 1309-37-1		5 R				10* *Fume				5* *Dust and fume, as Fe				with the exception of Iron oxides which are not biologically available							IARC-3 MAK-3B TLV-A4
Iron pentacarbonyl 13463-40-6	0.1	0.23	0.2	0.45					0.1*	0.23* *as Fe	0.2*	0.45*	0.1	0.81	I (2) Skin; D						
Iron salts, soluble, as Fe		1								1											
Iron sorbitol-citric acid complex 1338-16-5																					IARC-3
Isatidine 15503-86-3																					IARC-3
Isoamyl alcohol 123-51-3	100	361	125	452	100*	360* *primary and secondary			100*	360* *primary and secondary	125*	450*	20	73	I (4) C						

SUBSTANCE	ACGIH® TLVs®				OSHA PELs				NIOSH RELs				DFG MAKs				AIHA WEELs				CARCINOGENICITY CATEGORY
	TWA		STEL/CEIL(C)		TWA		STEL/CEIL(C)		TWA		STEL/CEIL(C)		TWA		PEAK/CEIL(C)		TWA		STEL/CEIL(C)		
CAS#	ppm	mg/m³	ppm	mg/m³	ppm	mg/m³	ppm	mg/m³	ppm	mg/m³	ppm	mg/m³	ppm	mg/m³	ppm	mg/m³	ppm	mg/m³	ppm	mg/m³	
Isobutanol (Isobutyl alcohol) 78-83-1	50	152			100	300			50	150			100	310	I (1) C						
Isobutyl acetate 110-19-0	150	713			150	700			150	700			100	480	I (2) C						
Isobutylamine 78-81-9													2	6.1	I (2) C 10 C 30 C						
Isobutyl nitrite 542-56-3		BEI$_M$	C 1 **IFV** C 4.2 **IFV**																		TLV-A3
Isobutyraldehyde 78-84-2																	25				
Isobutyronitrile 78-82-0									8	22											
Isocyanuric acid 108-80-5																	10* 5 **R** *Total dust				
Isoeugenol and its isomers 97-54-1; 5912-86-7; 5932-68-3														Sh							
Isonicotinic acid hydrazine (Isoniazid) 54-85-3																					IARC-3

SUBSTANCE / CAS#	ACGIH® TLVs® TWA ppm	mg/m³	STEL/CEIL(C) ppm	mg/m³	OSHA PELs TWA ppm	mg/m³	STEL/CEIL(C) ppm	mg/m³	NIOSH RELs TWA ppm	mg/m³	STEL/CEIL(C) ppm	mg/m³	DFG MAKs TWA ppm	mg/m³	PEAK/CEIL(C) ppm	mg/m³	AIHA WEELs TWA ppm	mg/m³	STEL/CEIL(C) ppm	mg/m³	CARCINOGENICITY CATEGORY
Isooctyl acrylate (2-Propenoic acid, isooctyl ester) 29590-42-9																	5				
Isooctyl alcohol 26952-21-6	50	266		Skin					50	270		Skin									
Isopentyl acetate (Isoamyl acetate) 123-92-2	50	266	100	532	100	525			100	525			50	270	I (1) D						
Isophorone 78-59-1			C 5	C 28	25	140			4	23			2	11	I (2) C						EPA-C MAK-3B TLV-A3
Isophorone diisocyanate 4098-71-9	0.005	0.045						Skin	0.005	0.045	0.02	0.18	0.005	0.046	I (1) C 0.01 C 0.092 Sah; D						
Isophosphamide 3778-73-2																					IARC-3
Isoprene 78-79-5													3	8.5	II (8) C; 5		2				IARC-2B MAK-5 NTP-R
Isopropenyl acetate 108-22-5													10	46	I (2) D						
2-Isopropoxyethanol (Ethylene glycol isopropyl ether) 109-59-1	25	106		Skin									5	22	II (8) Skin; C						

SUBSTANCE / CAS#	ACGIH® TLVs® TWA ppm	mg/m³	STEL/CEIL(C) ppm	mg/m³	OSHA PELs TWA ppm	mg/m³	STEL/CEIL(C) ppm	mg/m³	NIOSH RELs TWA ppm	mg/m³	STEL/CEIL(C) ppm	mg/m³	DFG MAKs TWA ppm	mg/m³	PEAK/CEIL(C) ppm	mg/m³	AIHA WEELs TWA ppm	mg/m³	STEL/CEIL(C) ppm	mg/m³	CARCINOGENICITY CATEGORY
Isopropyl acetate 108-21-4	100	418	200	836	250	950							100	420	I (2) C						
Isopropylamine 75-31-0	5	12	10	24	5	12							5	12	I (2) C 10 C 25 C						
N-Isopropylaniline 768-52-5	2	11 Skin; BEI_M							2	10 Skin											
Isopropyl ether 108-20-3	250	1040	310	1300	500	2100			500	2100			200	850	I (2) C						
Isopropyl glycidyl ether (IGE) 4016-14-2	50	238	75	356	50	240					C 50*	C 240* *15-min									MAK-3B
Isopropyl methyl phosphonic acid (IMPA) 1832-54-8																					EPA-D
Isopropyl oil (residue of Isopropyl alcohol production)																					IARC-3 MAK-3B
4-Isopropylphenyl isocyanate 31027-31-3														Sh							
N-Isopropyl-N'-phenyl-p-phenylenediamine 101-72-4													2 I	Sh; C	II (2)						

SUBSTANCE / CAS#	ACGIH® TLVs® TWA ppm	TWA mg/m³	STEL/CEIL(C) ppm	STEL/CEIL(C) mg/m³	OSHA PELs TWA ppm	TWA mg/m³	STEL/CEIL(C) ppm	STEL/CEIL(C) mg/m³	NIOSH RELs TWA ppm	TWA mg/m³	STEL/CEIL(C) ppm	STEL/CEIL(C) mg/m³	DFG MAKs TWA ppm	TWA mg/m³	PEAK/CEIL(C) ppm	PEAK/CEIL(C) mg/m³	AIHA WEELs TWA ppm	TWA mg/m³	STEL/CEIL(C) ppm	STEL/CEIL(C) mg/m³	CARCINOGENICITY CATEGORY
Isosafrole 120-58-1																					IARC-3
Isoxaben 82558-50-7																					EPA-C
Jacobine 6870-67-3																					IARC-3
Kaolin 1332-58-7		2 R E			15*; 5**			*Total dust **Respirable fraction	10*; 5**			*Total dust **Respirable fraction									MAK-3B* TLV-A4 *Quartz content must be considered separately
Kempferol 520-18-3																					IARC-3
Kerosene/Jet fuels as total hydrocarbon vapor 8008-20-6; 64742-81-0	200 Skin; P								100 Kerosene only												IARC-3* TLV-A3 *Jet fuels only
Ketene 463-51-4	0.5	0.86	1.5	2.6	0.5	0.9			0.5	0.9	1.5	3									
Kevlar 49 (p-Aramid fibrils) 24938-64-5																					IARC-3
Kojic acid 501-30-4																					IARC-3

SUBSTANCE CAS#	ACGIH® TLVs® TWA ppm	TWA mg/m³	STEL/CEIL(C) ppm	STEL/CEIL(C) mg/m³	OSHA PELs TWA ppm	TWA mg/m³	STEL/CEIL(C) ppm	STEL/CEIL(C) mg/m³	NIOSH RELs TWA ppm	TWA mg/m³	STEL/CEIL(C) ppm	STEL/CEIL(C) mg/m³	DFG MAKs TWA ppm	TWA mg/m³	PEAK/CEIL(C) ppm	PEAK/CEIL(C) mg/m³	AIHA WEELs TWA ppm	TWA mg/m³	STEL/CEIL(C) ppm	STEL/CEIL(C) mg/m³	CARCINOGENICITY CATEGORY
Lasiocarpine 303-34-4																					IARC-2B
Lauric acid 143-07-7																					MAK-3A
Lauroyl peroxide 105-74-8																					IARC-3
Lead [7439-92-1] and inorganic compounds, as Pb	0.05	BEI			0.05 including organic Lead soaps *See* 29 CFR 1910.1025				0.05* *8-hr TWA excluding Lead arsenate *See* Pocket Guide App. C				except Lead arsenate and Lead chromate; as Inhalable fraction 3A								EPA-B2 NTP-R IARC-2A*; 2B TLV-A3 MAK-2 *inorganic compounds
Lead, organic compounds					for organic Lead soaps, *see* Lead and inorganic compounds, as Pb																IARC-3
Lead arsenate 3687-31-8	TLV® withdrawn due to insufficient data				0.01* *as As *See* 29 CFR 1910.1018				*See* Arsenic and inorganic compounds				as As 3A								EPA-B2 NTP-R IARC-1; 2A OSHA-Ca MAK-1
Lead chromate 7758-97-6	0.05* 0.012** *as Pb; BEI **as Cr								*See* Chromium (VI) inorganic compounds, insoluble				*See* Chromium (VI) inorganic compounds, insoluble								EPA*-A**; TLV-A2 D***; CBD**; K** NTP-K* *as Cr (VI) **inhalation ***oral
Lead chromate oxide 18454-12-1													*See* Chromium (VI) inorganic compounds, insoluble								

SUBSTANCE / CAS#	ACGIH® TLVs® TWA ppm	mg/m³	STEL/CEIL(C) ppm	mg/m³	OSHA PELs TWA ppm	mg/m³	STEL/CEIL(C) ppm	mg/m³	NIOSH RELs TWA ppm	mg/m³	STEL/CEIL(C) ppm	mg/m³	DFG MAKs TWA ppm	mg/m³	PEAK/CEIL(C) ppm	mg/m³	AIHA WEELs TWA ppm	mg/m³	STEL/CEIL(C) ppm	mg/m³	CARCINOGENICITY CATEGORY
Lead phosphate 7446-27-7	*See* Lead and inorganic compounds, as Pb				0.05				*See* Lead and inorganic compounds												EPA-B2 IARC-2A NTP-R TLV-A3
					See 29 CFR 1910.1025																
Levofuraltadone (5-[Morpholinomethyl]-3-[(5-nitrofurfurylidene) amino]-2-oxazolidinone) 3795-88-8																					IARC-2B
Light Green SF 5141-20-8																					IARC-3
D-Limonene 5989-27-5													5	28	II (4)						IARC-3
													Skin; Sh; C								
DL-Limonene 138-86-3													and similar mixtures Sh				30				
L-Limonene (β-Limonene) 5989-54-8													Sh								
Lindane (γ-Hexachloro-cyclohexane) 58-89-9	0.5				0.5				0.5				0.1 I		II (8)						MAK-4 TLV-A3 NTP-R* *and other HCH isomers
	Skin				Skin				Skin				Skin; C								
Linuron 330-55-2																					EPA-C

SUBSTANCE / CAS#	ACGIH® TLVs® TWA ppm	TWA mg/m³	STEL/CEIL(C) ppm	mg/m³	OSHA PELs TWA ppm	mg/m³	STEL/CEIL(C) ppm	mg/m³	NIOSH RELs TWA ppm	mg/m³	STEL/CEIL(C) ppm	mg/m³	DFG MAKs TWA ppm	mg/m³	PEAK/CEIL(C) ppm	mg/m³	AIHA WEELs TWA ppm	mg/m³	STEL/CEIL(C) ppm	mg/m³	CARCINOGENICITY CATEGORY
Lithium hydride 7580-67-8		0.025				0.025				0.025											
Lithium hydroxide 1310-65-2																				C 1	
Lithium oxide 12057-24-8																				C 1	
L.P.G. (Liquefied petroleum gas) 68476-85-7	Refer to Appendix F: Minimal Oxygen Content				1000	1800			1000	1800											
Luteoskyrin 21884-44-6																					IARC-3
Magenta 632-99-5																					IARC-1*; 2B *production
Magnesite 546-93-0	TLV® withdrawn due to insufficient data				15*; 5** *Total dust **Respirable fraction				10*; 5** *Total dust **Respirable fraction												
Magnesium oxide 1309-48-4		10 I				15* Fume *Total particulate								4 I 1.5 R C							TLV-A4
Magnesium oxide sulfate, fibrous dust 12286-12-3																					MAK-3B

SUBSTANCE / CAS#	ACGIH® TLVs® TWA ppm	mg/m³	STEL/CEIL(C) ppm	mg/m³	OSHA PELs TWA ppm	mg/m³	STEL/CEIL(C) ppm	mg/m³	NIOSH RELs TWA ppm	mg/m³	STEL/CEIL(C) ppm	mg/m³	DFG MAKs TWA ppm	mg/m³	PEAK/CEIL(C) ppm	mg/m³	AIHA WEELs TWA ppm	mg/m³	STEL/CEIL(C) ppm	mg/m³	CARCINOGENICITY CATEGORY
Malathion 121-75-5	1 **IFV** Skin; BEI_A				15* *Total dust Skin				10 Skin				15 **I** D		II (4)						IARC-3 TLV-A4
Maleic anhydride 108-31-6	0.0025* *IFV (SEN) NIC-DSEN; RSEN	0.01*			0.25	1			0.25	1			0.1 Sah; C	0.41	I (1) C 0.2 C 0.81						TLV-A4
Maleic hydrazide 123-33-1																					IARC-3
Malonaldehyde 542-78-9									*See* Pocket Guide Apps. A and C												IARC-3 NIOSH-Ca
Malononitrile 109-77-3									3	8											
Mancozeb 8018-01-7																	1 DSEN				
Manganese [7439-96-5] **and inorganic compounds, as Mn**	0.02 **R** 0.1 **I**						C 5		1	3			0.2 **I** 0.02 **R** C		II (8) II (1)* *Permanganates only						EPA-D TLV-A4
Manganese, fume, as Mn 7439-96-5	0.2						C 5		1	3			0.2 **I** 0.02 **R** C		II (8)						EPA-D
Manganese cyclopenta-dienyl tricarbonyl, as Mn 12079-65-1	0.1 Skin						C 5		0.1 Skin				0.2 **I** 0.02 **R** C		II (8)						

SUBSTANCE CAS#	ACGIH® TLVs® TWA ppm	mg/m³	STEL/CEIL(C) ppm	mg/m³	OSHA PELs TWA ppm	mg/m³	STEL/CEIL(C) ppm	mg/m³	NIOSH RELs TWA ppm	mg/m³	STEL/CEIL(C) ppm	mg/m³	DFG MAKs TWA ppm	mg/m³	PEAK/CEIL(C) ppm	mg/m³	AIHA WEELs TWA ppm	mg/m³	STEL/CEIL(C) ppm	mg/m³	CARCINOGENICITY CATEGORY
Manganous ethylenebis-(dithiocarbamate) (Maneb) 12427-38-2														Sh							IARC-3
Mannomustine dihydrochloride 551-74-6																					IARC-3
Mate, absolute (Tea oil) 68916-96-1																					IARC-3
Medphalan 13045-94-8																					IARC-3
Medroxyprogesterone acetate 71-58-9																					IARC-2B
Melamine 108-78-1																		10 I 5 R			IARC-3
Melphalan 148-82-3																					IARC-1 NTP-K
Merbromin 129-16-8														Sh							
2-Mercaptobenzo-thiazole 149-30-4														4 I 1.5 R Sh; C				5 Skin; DSEN			MAK-3B

SUBSTANCE / CAS#	ACGIH® TLVs® TWA ppm	mg/m³	STEL/CEIL(C) ppm	mg/m³	OSHA PELs TWA ppm	mg/m³	STEL/CEIL(C) ppm	mg/m³	NIOSH RELs TWA ppm	mg/m³	STEL/CEIL(C) ppm	mg/m³	DFG MAKs TWA ppm	mg/m³	PEAK/CEIL(C) ppm	mg/m³	AIHA WEELs TWA ppm	mg/m³	STEL/CEIL(C) ppm	mg/m³	CARCINOGENICITY CATEGORY
Mercaptoethanol 60-24-2																	0.2		Skin		
6-Mercaptopurine 50-44-2																					IARC-3
Mercuric chloride 7487-94-7																					EPA-C
Mercury, alkyl compounds, as Hg	0.01			0.03	0.01		C 0.04		0.01			0.03									MAK-3B
		Skin								Skin				Skin; Sh							
Mercury, aryl compounds, as Hg 7439-97-6	0.1				0.1						C 0.1										MAK-3B
		Skin				*See OSHA standard interpretation memo*				Skin				Skin; Sh							
Mercury, elemental and inorganic compounds, as Hg 7439-97-6	0.025				0.1				0.05*		C 0.1		0.02 **I**		II (8)						EPA-D IARC-3 MAK-3B TLV-A4
		Skin; BEI				*See OSHA standard interpretation memo*			*Vapor Skin				Skin; Sh; D							
Merphalan 531-76-0																					IARC-2B
Mesityl oxide 141-79-7	15	60	25	100	25	100			10	40			5	20	I (2)						
														Skin; D							
Metabisulfites 23134-05-6																					IARC-3

SUBSTANCE / CAS#	ACGIH® TLVs® TWA ppm	mg/m³	STEL/CEIL(C) ppm	mg/m³	OSHA PELs TWA ppm	mg/m³	STEL/CEIL(C) ppm	mg/m³	NIOSH RELs TWA ppm	mg/m³	STEL/CEIL(C) ppm	mg/m³	DFG MAKs TWA ppm	mg/m³	PEAK/CEIL(C) ppm	mg/m³	AIHA WEELs TWA ppm	mg/m³	STEL/CEIL(C) ppm	mg/m³	CARCINOGENICITY CATEGORY
Metal-working fluids (capable of yielding nitrosamines)																					MAK-3B
Methacrylic acid 79-41-4	20	70							20	70 Skin			5	18 C	I (2)						
Methane 74-82-8	Refer to Appendix F: Minimal Oxygen Content																				
Methanol (Methyl alcohol) 67-56-1	200	262 Skin; BEI	250	328	200	260			200	260 Skin	250	325	200	270 Skin; C	II (4)						
Methenamin 3-chlor-allylchloride 4080-31-3													2 I releases Formaldehyde Sh; B		II (2)						
Methidathion 950-37-8																					EPA-C
Methimazole 60-56-0																					IARC-3
Methomyl 16752-77-5	(2.5) NIC-0.2 **IFV** NIC-Skin	BEI_A							2.5												TLV-A4
Methotrexate 59-05-2																					IARC-3

SUBSTANCE / CAS#	ACGIH® TLVs® TWA ppm	mg/m³	STEL/CEIL(C) ppm	mg/m³	OSHA PELs TWA ppm	mg/m³	STEL/CEIL(C) ppm	mg/m³	NIOSH RELs TWA ppm	mg/m³	STEL/CEIL(C) ppm	mg/m³	DFG MAKs TWA ppm	mg/m³	PEAK/CEIL(C) ppm	mg/m³	AIHA WEELs TWA ppm	mg/m³	STEL/CEIL(C) ppm	mg/m³	CARCINOGENICITY CATEGORY
Methoxyacetic acid 625-45-6													1	3.7	II (8)						
													Skin; B								
Methoxychlor 72-43-5		10				15*								15 **I**	II (8)						EPA-D IARC-3 NIOSH-Ca TLV-A4
					*Total dust				*See* Pocket Guide App. A				D								
2-Methoxyethanol (EGME) 109-86-4	0.1	0.3			25	80			0.1	0.3			1*	3.2	II (8)						
	Skin; BEI				Skin				Skin				*sum of the concentrations of EGME and its acetate in air Skin; B				Skin; B				
2-Methoxyethyl acetate (EGMEA) 110-49-6	0.1	0.5			25	120			0.1	0.5			1*	4.9	II (8)						
	Skin; BEI				Skin				Skin				*sum of the concentrations of EGME and its acetate in air Skin; B				Skin; B				
Methoxyflurane 76-38-0											C 2*	C 13.5*									
									*60-min; for exposure to waste anesthetic gases											
(2-Methoxymethylethoxy)-propanol (DPGME) 34590-94-8	100	606	150	909	100	600			100	600	150	900	50	310	I (1)						
	Skin				Skin				Skin				D								
4-Methoxyphenol 150-76-5	5								5												
1-Methoxy-2-propanol (Propylene glycol monomethyl ether; PGME) 107-98-2	50	184	100	369					100	360	150	540	100	370	I (2)						TLV-A4
													C								
2-Methoxy-1-propanol (Propylene glycol 2-methyl ether) 1589-47-5													5	19	II (8)						
													Skin; B								

SUBSTANCE / CAS#	ACGIH® TLVs® TWA ppm	mg/m³	STEL/CEIL(C) ppm	mg/m³	OSHA PELs TWA ppm	mg/m³	STEL/CEIL(C) ppm	mg/m³	NIOSH RELs TWA ppm	mg/m³	STEL/CEIL(C) ppm	mg/m³	DFG MAKs TWA ppm	mg/m³	PEAK/CEIL(C) ppm	mg/m³	AIHA WEELs TWA ppm	mg/m³	STEL/CEIL(C) ppm	mg/m³	CARCINOGENICITY CATEGORY
1-Methoxypropyl-2-acetate (Propylene glycol mono-methyl ether acetate) 108-65-6													50	270	I (1) C		50				
2-Methoxypropyl-1-acetate (Propylene glycol 2-methyl ether-1-acetate) 70657-70-4													5	28	II (8) Skin; B						
3-Methoxypropylamine 5332-73-0																	5		15		
5-Methoxypsoralen 484-20-8																					IARC-2A
8-Methoxypsoralen (Methoxsalen) plus ultra-violet A radiation 298-81-7																					IARC-1 NTP-K
Methyl acetate 79-20-9	200	606	250	757	200	610			200	610	250	760	100	310	I (4) C						
Methyl acetylene (Propyne) 74-99-7	1000	1640			1000	1650			1000	1650											
Methyl acetylene-propadiene mixture (MAPP)	1000	1640	1250	2050	1000	1800			1000	1800	1250	2250									
Methyl acrylate (Acrylic acid, methyl ester) 96-33-3	2	7			10	35			10	35			5	18	I (1)						EPA-D IARC-3 TLV-A4
	Skin; (SEN) NIC-DSEN				Skin				Skin				Sh; D								

SUBSTANCE / CAS#	ACGIH® TLVs® TWA ppm	mg/m³	STEL/CEIL(C) ppm	mg/m³	OSHA PELs TWA ppm	mg/m³	STEL/CEIL(C) ppm	mg/m³	NIOSH RELs TWA ppm	mg/m³	STEL/CEIL(C) ppm	mg/m³	DFG MAKs TWA ppm	mg/m³	PEAK/CEIL(C) ppm	mg/m³	AIHA WEELs TWA ppm	mg/m³	STEL/CEIL(C) ppm	mg/m³	CARCINOGENICITY CATEGORY
Methylacrylonitrile 126-98-7	1	2.7		Skin					1	3		Skin									TLV-A4
Methylal (Dimethoxymethane) 109-87-5	1000	3110			1000	3100			1000	3100			1000	3200	II (2) C						
Methylamine 74-89-5	5	6.4	15	19	10	12			10	12			10	13	I (1) C 10 D	C 13					
Methyl n-amyl ketone (2-Heptanone) 110-43-0	50	233			100	465			100	465											
5-Methylangelicin plus ultraviolet A radiation 73459-03-7																					IARC-3
N-Methyl aniline (Monomethyl aniline) 100-61-8	0.5	2.2		Skin; BEI$_M$	2	9		Skin	0.5	2		Skin	0.5	2.2	II (2) Skin; D						
Methylarsonic acid 124-58-3																					IARC-2B
tris(2-Methyl-1-aziridi-nyl)phosphine oxide 57-39-6																					IARC-3
Methylazoxymethanol acetate 592-62-1																					IARC-2B

SUBSTANCE	ACGIH® TLVs®				OSHA PELs				NIOSH RELs				DFG MAKs				AIHA WEELs				CARCINOGENICITY CATEGORY
	TWA		STEL/CEIL(C)		TWA		STEL/CEIL(C)		TWA		STEL/CEIL(C)		TWA		PEAK/CEIL(C)		TWA		STEL/CEIL(C)		
CAS#	ppm	mg/m³	ppm	mg/m³	ppm	mg/m³	ppm	mg/m³	ppm	mg/m³	ppm	mg/m³	ppm	mg/m³	ppm	mg/m³	ppm	mg/m³	ppm	mg/m³	
Methyl bromide 74-83-9	1	3.9					C 20	C 80					1	3.9	I (2)						EPA-D TLV-A4 IARC-3 MAK-3B NIOSH-Ca
		Skin				Skin			*See* Pocket Guide App. A					D							
2-Methylbutyl acetate 624-41-9	50	266	100	532									50	270	I (1)						
														C							
Methyl tert-butyl ether (MTBE) 1634-04-4	50	180											50	180	I (1.5)						IARC-3 MAK-3B TLV-A3
														C							
Methyl n-butyl ketone (2-Hexanone) 591-78-6	5	20	10	40	100	410			1	4			5	21	II (8)						EPA-I
		Skin; BEI												Skin						
Methyl carbamate 598-55-0																					IARC-3
Methyl chloride 74-87-3	50	103	100	207	100		C 200; 300*						50	100	II (2)						EPA-D NIOSH-Ca CBD TLV-A4 IARC-3 MAK-3B
		Skin				*5-min peak in any 3 hrs			*See* Pocket Guide App. A					Skin; B						
Methyl chloroform (1,1,1-Trichloroethane) 71-55-6	350	1910	450	2460	350	1900					C 350* *15-min	C 1900*	200	1100	II (1)						EPA-II IARC-3 TLV-A4
		BEI							*See* Pocket Guide App. C					Skin; C						
Methyl chloroformate (Chloroformic acid methyl ester) 79-22-1													0.2	0.78	I (2)						
														C							
1-Methylchrysene 3351-28-8																					IARC-3

SUBSTANCE / CAS#	ACGIH® TLVs® TWA ppm	ACGIH® TLVs® TWA mg/m³	ACGIH® TLVs® STEL/CEIL(C) ppm	ACGIH® TLVs® STEL/CEIL(C) mg/m³	OSHA PELs TWA ppm	OSHA PELs TWA mg/m³	OSHA PELs STEL/CEIL(C) ppm	OSHA PELs STEL/CEIL(C) mg/m³	NIOSH RELs TWA ppm	NIOSH RELs TWA mg/m³	NIOSH RELs STEL/CEIL(C) ppm	NIOSH RELs STEL/CEIL(C) mg/m³	DFG MAKs TWA ppm	DFG MAKs TWA mg/m³	DFG MAKs PEAK/CEIL(C) ppm	DFG MAKs PEAK/CEIL(C) mg/m³	AIHA WEELs TWA ppm	AIHA WEELs TWA mg/m³	AIHA WEELs STEL/CEIL(C) ppm	AIHA WEELs STEL/CEIL(C) mg/m³	CARCINOGENICITY CATEGORY
2-Methylchrysene 3351-32-4																					IARC-3
3-Methylchrysene 3351-31-3																					IARC-3
4-Methylchrysene 3351-30-2																					IARC-3
5-Methylchrysene 3697-24-3																					IARC-2B NTP-R
6-Methylchrysene 1705-85-7																					IARC-3
Methyl-2-cyano-acrylate 137-05-3	0.2	1							2	8	4	16	2	9.2	I (1) D						
Methylcyclohexane 108-87-2	400	1610			500	2000			400	1600			200	810	II (2) D						
Methylcyclohexanol 25639-42-3	50	234			100	470			50	235											
o-Methylcyclohexanone 583-60-8	50	229	75	344	100	460			50	230	75	345									

ACGIH: Skin   OSHA: Skin   NIOSH: Skin

SUBSTANCE / CAS#	ACGIH® TLVs® TWA ppm	mg/m³	STEL/CEIL(C) ppm	mg/m³	OSHA PELs TWA ppm	mg/m³	STEL/CEIL(C) ppm	mg/m³	NIOSH RELs TWA ppm	mg/m³	STEL/CEIL(C) ppm	mg/m³	DFG MAKs TWA ppm	mg/m³	PEAK/CEIL(C) ppm	mg/m³	AIHA WEELs TWA ppm	mg/m³	STEL/CEIL(C) ppm	mg/m³	CARCINOGENICITY CATEGORY
2-Methylcyclopentadienyl manganese tricarbonyl, as Mn 12108-13-3		0.2								0.2											
	Skin									Skin											
Methyl demeton (Demeton-methyl) 8022-00-2		0.05 IFV								0.5			0.5	4.8	II (2)						
	Skin; BEI$_A$									Skin			Skin								
N-Methyl-N,4-dinitroso-aniline 99-80-9																					IARC-3
Methylene bisphenyl iso-cyanate (MDI; Diphenylmethane-4,4'-diisocyanate) 101-68-8	0.005	0.051					C 0.02	C 0.2	0.005	0.05	C 0.02*	C 0.2*		0.05 I	I (1) C 0.1						EPA-CBD; D IARC-3 MAK-4
											*10-min		Skin; Sah; C								
4,4'-Methylene bis(2-chloroaniline) (MBOCA) 101-14-4	0.01	0.11							0.003												IARC-1 TLV-A2 MAK-2 NIOSH-Ca NTP-R
	Skin; BEI								Skin See Pocket Guide App. A				Skin								
Methylene bis(4-cyclo-hexylisocyanate) 5124-30-1	0.005	0.054									C 0.01	C 0.11									
4,4'-Methylene dianiline (4,4'-Diaminodiphenyl-methane) 101-77-9	0.1	0.81			0.01		0.1														IARC-2B NTP-R* MAK-2 OSHA-Ca NIOSH-Ca TLV-A3
	Skin				See 29 CFR 1910.1050				See Pocket Guide App. A				Skin; Sh								*and its salts; CAS: 13552-44-8
4,4'-Methylene bis(N,N'-dimethyl)aniline (Michler's base) 101-61-1																					EPA-B2 IARC-2B MAK-2 NTP-R
4,4'-Methylene bis-(2-methylaniline) 838-88-0																					IARC-2B MAK-2
													Skin								

SUBSTANCE / CAS#	ACGIH® TLVs® TWA ppm	mg/m³	STEL/CEIL(C) ppm	mg/m³	OSHA PELs TWA ppm	mg/m³	STEL/CEIL(C) ppm	mg/m³	NIOSH RELs TWA ppm	mg/m³	STEL/CEIL(C) ppm	mg/m³	DFG MAKs TWA ppm	mg/m³	PEAK/CEIL(C) ppm	mg/m³	AIHA WEELs TWA ppm	mg/m³	STEL/CEIL(C) ppm	mg/m³	CARCINOGENICITY CATEGORY
N,N′-Methylene-bis-(5-methyloxazolidine) 66204-44-2														Sh							
Methyl ethyl ketone (MEK; 2-Butanone) 78-93-3	200	590 BEI	300	885	200	590			200	590	300	885	200	600 Skin; C	I (1)						EPA-I
Methyl ethyl ketone peroxide 1338-23-4			C 0.2	C 1.5							C 0.2	C 1.5									
Methyl ethyl ketoxime (2-Butanone oxime) 96-29-7														Skin; Sh			10	DSEN			MAK-2
Methyleugenol 93-15-2																					IARC-2B NTP-R
Methyl formate (Formic acid methyl ester) 107-31-3	(100) NIC-50	(246) NIC-123 NIC-Skin	150	368	100	250			100	250	150	375	50	120 Skin; C	II (4)						
2-Methylfluoranthene 33543-31-6																					IARC-3
3-Methylfluoranthene 1706-01-0																					IARC-3
Methylglyoxal 78-98-8																					IARC-3

SUBSTANCE CAS#	ACGIH® TLVs® TWA ppm	TWA mg/m³	STEL/CEIL(C) ppm	mg/m³	OSHA PELs TWA ppm	TWA mg/m³	STEL/CEIL(C) ppm	mg/m³	NIOSH RELs TWA ppm	TWA mg/m³	STEL/CEIL(C) ppm	mg/m³	DFG MAKs TWA ppm	TWA mg/m³	PEAK/CEIL(C) ppm	mg/m³	AIHA WEELs TWA ppm	TWA mg/m³	STEL/CEIL(C) ppm	mg/m³	CARCINOGENICITY CATEGORY
Methyl hydrazine (Monomethyl hydrazine) 60-34-4	0.01	0.019					C 0.2	C 0.35			C 0.04*	C 0.08* *120-min									NIOSH-Ca TLV-A3
		Skin				Skin			*See* Pocket Guide App. A				Skin; Sh								
2-Methylimidazole 693-98-1																					IARC-2B
4-Methylimidazole 822-36-6																					IARC-2B
Methyl iodide 74-88-4	2	12			5	28			2	10 Skin *See* Pocket Guide App. A			Skin								IARC-3 MAK-2 NIOSH-Ca
		Skin				Skin															
Methyl isoamyl ketone (Methyl-2-hexanone) 110-12-3	20	93	50	233	100	475			50	240			10	47 D	I (2)						
Methyl isobutyl carbinol (Methyl amyl alcohol; 4-Methyl-2-pentanol) 108-11-2	25	104	40	167	25	100			25	100	40	165	20	85 D	I (1)						
		Skin				Skin				Skin											
Methyl isobutyl ketone (Hexone) 108-10-1	20	82	75	307	100	410			50	205	75	300	20	83	I (2)						EPA-I IARC-2B TLV-A3
		BEI											Skin; C							
Methyl isocyanate 624-83-9	0.02	0.047	NIC-0.06	NIC-0.14	0.02	0.05			0.02	0.05			0.01	0.024	I (1)						
	Skin; NIC-DSEN					Skin				Skin				D						
Methyl isopropyl ketone (MIPK) 563-80-4	20	70							200	705											

SUBSTANCE CAS#	ACGIH® TLVs TWA ppm	mg/m³	STEL/CEIL(C) ppm	mg/m³	OSHA PELs TWA ppm	mg/m³	STEL/CEIL(C) ppm	mg/m³	NIOSH RELs TWA ppm	mg/m³	STEL/CEIL(C) ppm	mg/m³	DFG MAKs TWA ppm	mg/m³	PEAK/CEIL(C) ppm	mg/m³	AIHA WEELs TWA ppm	mg/m³	STEL/CEIL(C) ppm	mg/m³	CARCINOGENICITY CATEGORY
2-Methyl-4-isothiazolin-3-one 2682-20-4														Sh							
Methyl mercaptan (Methanethiol) 74-93-1	0.5	0.98					C 10	C 20			C 0.5*	C 1* *15-min	0.5	1 D	II (2)						
Methyl mercury 22967-92-6					0.01*		C 0.04* *as Hg		See Mercury, alkyl compounds				Skin; Sh								EPA-C IARC-2B* MAK-3B *compounds
Methyl methacrylate (Methacrylic acid methyl ester) 80-62-6	50	205 (SEN) NIC-DSEN; RSEN	100	410	100	410			100	410			50	210 Sh; C	I (2)						EPA-NL; E IARC-3 TLV-A4
Methyl methanesulfonate 66-27-3																					IARC-2A NTP-R
1-Methyl naphthalene [90-12-0] and 2-Methyl naphthalene [91-57-6]	0.5	3 Skin																			EPA-I* TLV-A4 *CAS: 91-57-6 only
2-Methyl-1-nitroanthra-quinone, uncertain purity 129-15-7																					IARC-2B
N-Methyl-N′-nitro-N-nitrosoguanidine (MNNG) 70-25-7																					IARC-2A NTP-R
3-(Methylnitrosamino) propionitrile (3-[N-Nitro-somethylamino]pro-pionitrile) 60153-49-3																					IARC-2B

SUBSTANCE CAS#	ACGIH® TLVs® TWA ppm	ACGIH® TLVs® TWA mg/m³	ACGIH® TLVs® STEL/CEIL(C) ppm	ACGIH® TLVs® STEL/CEIL(C) mg/m³	OSHA PELs TWA ppm	OSHA PELs TWA mg/m³	OSHA PELs STEL/CEIL(C) ppm	OSHA PELs STEL/CEIL(C) mg/m³	NIOSH RELs TWA ppm	NIOSH RELs TWA mg/m³	NIOSH RELs STEL/CEIL(C) ppm	NIOSH RELs STEL/CEIL(C) mg/m³	DFG MAKs TWA ppm	DFG MAKs TWA mg/m³	DFG MAKs PEAK/CEIL(C) ppm	DFG MAKs PEAK/CEIL(C) mg/m³	AIHA WEELs TWA ppm	AIHA WEELs TWA mg/m³	AIHA WEELs STEL/CEIL(C) ppm	AIHA WEELs STEL/CEIL(C) mg/m³	CARCINOGENICITY CATEGORY
N-Methyl-N-nitrosour-ethane 615-53-2																					IARC-2B
N-Methylolacrylamide 90456-67-0																					IARC-3
Methyl parathion 298-00-0	0.02 IFV Skin; BEI_A								0.2 Skin												IARC-3 TLV-A4
2-Methylphenanthrene 832-69-9																					IARC-3
Methyl propyl ketone (2-Pentanone) 107-87-9		150	529		200	700			150	530											
1-Methylpyrene 2381-21-7														Skin							MAK-2
7-Methylpyrido[3,4-c]-psoralen 85878-63-3																					IARC-3
N-Methyl-2-pyrrolidone 872-50-4													20	82 Vapor Skin; C	II (2)		10		Skin		
Methyl Red 493-52-7																					IARC-3

SUBSTANCE CAS#	ACGIH® TLVs® TWA ppm	ACGIH® TLVs® TWA mg/m³	ACGIH® TLVs® STEL/CEIL(C) ppm	ACGIH® TLVs® STEL/CEIL(C) mg/m³	OSHA PELs TWA ppm	OSHA PELs TWA mg/m³	OSHA PELs STEL/CEIL(C) ppm	OSHA PELs STEL/CEIL(C) mg/m³	NIOSH RELs TWA ppm	NIOSH RELs TWA mg/m³	NIOSH RELs STEL/CEIL(C) ppm	NIOSH RELs STEL/CEIL(C) mg/m³	DFG MAKs TWA ppm	DFG MAKs TWA mg/m³	DFG MAKs PEAK/CEIL(C) ppm	DFG MAKs PEAK/CEIL(C) mg/m³	AIHA WEELs TWA ppm	AIHA WEELs TWA mg/m³	AIHA WEELs STEL/CEIL(C) ppm	AIHA WEELs STEL/CEIL(C) mg/m³	CARCINOGENICITY CATEGORY
Methyl selenac 144-34-3																					IARC-3
Methyl silicate 681-84-5	1	6							1	6											
α-Methyl styrene 98-83-9	10	48					C 100	C 480	50	240	100	485	50	250	I (2) D						IARC-2B TLV-A3
Methyltetrahydrophthalic anhydride 11070-44-3															Sa						
Methylthiouracil 56-04-2																					IARC-2B
Methyltrichlorosilane 75-79-6																			C 1		
Methyl vinyl ether 107-25-5													200	480	II (2) C						
Methyl vinyl ketone (3-Buten-2-one) 78-94-4			C 0.2 Skin; SEN	C 0.6											Skin; Sh						
Metolachlor 51218-45-2																					EPA-C

SUBSTANCE / CAS#	ACGIH® TLVs® TWA ppm	TWA mg/m³	STEL/CEIL(C) ppm	mg/m³	OSHA PELs TWA ppm	TWA mg/m³	STEL/CEIL(C) ppm	mg/m³	NIOSH RELs TWA ppm	TWA mg/m³	STEL/CEIL(C) ppm	mg/m³	DFG MAKs TWA ppm	TWA mg/m³	PEAK/CEIL(C) ppm	mg/m³	AIHA WEELs TWA ppm	TWA mg/m³	STEL/CEIL(C) ppm	mg/m³	CARCINOGENICITY CATEGORY
Metribuzin 21087-64-9	5								5												EPA-D TLV-A4
Metronidazole 443-48-1																					IARC-2B NTP-R
Mevinphos 7786-34-7	0.01 IFV				0.1				0.01	0.1	0.03	0.3	0.01	0.093	II (2)						TLV-A4
	Skin; BEI_A				Skin				Skin				Skin								
Mica 12001-26-2		3 R			20 mppcf < 1% Crystalline silica					3* *Respirable dust; containing < 1% Quartz											
Michler's ketone 90-94-8																					IARC-2B MAK-2 NTP-R
Microbial rennets: endothiapepsin and mucorpepsin														Sa							
Microcystin-LR 101043-37-2																					IARC-2B
Mineral oil, Pure, highly and severely refined		5 I excluding Metal working fluids																			IARC-3* TLV-A4 *highly refined
Mineral oil, Poorly and mildly refined		excluding Metal working fluids L																			IARC-1* NTP-K TLV-A2 *untreated, mildly treated

SUBSTANCE / CAS#	ACGIH® TLVs® TWA ppm	mg/m³	STEL/CEIL(C) ppm	mg/m³	OSHA PELs TWA ppm	mg/m³	STEL/CEIL(C) ppm	mg/m³	NIOSH RELs TWA ppm	mg/m³	STEL/CEIL(C) ppm	mg/m³	DFG MAKs TWA ppm	mg/m³	PEAK/CEIL(C) ppm	mg/m³	AIHA WEELs TWA ppm	mg/m³	STEL/CEIL(C) ppm	mg/m³	CARCINOGENICITY CATEGORY
Mineral wool fiber	*See* Synthetic vitreous fibers									5*											
									*Total mineral wool dust, or 3 f/cc TWA (fibers ≤ 3.5 µm diam; ≥ 10 µm length)												
Mirex 2385-85-5																					IARC-2B NTP-R
Mitomycin C 50-07-7																					IARC-2B
Mitoxantrone 65271-80-9																					IARC-2B
Modacrylic fibers																					IARC-3
Molybdenum [7439-98-7] and insoluble compounds, as Mo		10 **I** 3 **R**			*15 *Total dust																
Molybdenum [7439-98-7] and soluble compounds, as Mo		0.5 **R**			5																TLV-A3
Molybdenum trioxide 1313-27-5																					MAK-3B
Monochloroacetic acid 79-11-8	0.5 **IFV** Skin		2 **IFV**														0.5 Skin				TLV-A4

SUBSTANCE CAS#	ACGIH® TLVs® TWA ppm	TWA mg/m³	STEL/CEIL(C) ppm	STEL/CEIL(C) mg/m³	OSHA PELs TWA ppm	TWA mg/m³	STEL/CEIL(C) ppm	STEL/CEIL(C) mg/m³	NIOSH RELs TWA ppm	TWA mg/m³	STEL/CEIL(C) ppm	STEL/CEIL(C) mg/m³	DFG MAKs TWA ppm	TWA mg/m³	PEAK/CEIL(C) ppm	PEAK/CEIL(C) mg/m³	AIHA WEELs TWA ppm	TWA mg/m³	STEL/CEIL(C) ppm	STEL/CEIL(C) mg/m³	CARCINOGENICITY CATEGORY
3-Monochloro-1,2-propanediol 96-24-2													0.005	0.025	II (8)						IARC-2B MAK-3B
													Skin; D								
Monocrotaline 315-22-0																					IARC-2B
Monocrotophos 6923-22-4	0.05 IFV								0.25												TLV-A4
		Skin; BEI_A																			
Mono-n-butyltin compounds, as Sn													0.004*	0.02 I	I (1)						MAK-4
													Skin**; C								
													*can also be found as vapor **for n-butyltin cmpds whose organic ligands are already designated "Sa" or "Sh", these designations also apply							
Mono-n-octyltin compounds, as Sn													0.002*	0.0098 I	II (2)						MAK-4
													Skin**; C								
													*can also be found as vapor **for n-octyltin cmpds whose organic ligands are already designated "Sa" or "Sh", these designations also apply							
Monuron 150-68-5																					IARC-3
Morpholine 110-91-8	20	71			20	70			20	70	30	105	10	36	I (2)						IARC-3 TLV-A4
		Skin				Skin				Skin				D							

SUBSTANCE / CAS#	ACGIH® TLVs® TWA ppm	mg/m³	STEL/CEIL(C) ppm	mg/m³	OSHA PELs TWA ppm	mg/m³	STEL/CEIL(C) ppm	mg/m³	NIOSH RELs TWA ppm	mg/m³	STEL/CEIL(C) ppm	mg/m³	DFG MAKs TWA ppm	mg/m³	PEAK/CEIL(C) ppm	mg/m³	AIHA WEELs TWA ppm	mg/m³	STEL/CEIL(C) ppm	mg/m³	CARCINOGENICITY CATEGORY
2-(4-Morpholinylmercapto)benzothiazole 102-77-2													Sh								
Musk ambrette 83-66-9																					IARC-3
Musk xylene 81-15-2																					IARC-3
Mustard gas (2,2′-Dichlorodiethyl sulfide) 505-60-2													Skin								IARC-1 MAK-1 NTP-K
Nafenopin 3771-19-5																					IARC-2B
Naled (Dibrom; Dimethyl-1,2-dibromo-2,2-dichloroethylphosphate) 300-76-5	0.1 IFV Skin; (SEN); BEI_A NIC-DSEN				3				3 Skin				1 I Skin; Sh; C		II (2)						TLV-A4
Naphtha, coal tar 8030-30-6					100	400			100	400											
Naphtha, petroleum, hydrotreated, heavy 64742-48-9													50 D	300	II (2)						
Naphthalene 91-20-3	10 Skin; BEI NIC-A3	52	(15)	(79)	10	50			10	50	15	75	Skin; 3B								EPA-CBD; C IARC-2B MAK-2 NTP-R (TLV-A4)

SUBSTANCE / CAS#	ACGIH® TLVs® TWA ppm	TWA mg/m³	STEL/CEIL(C) ppm	STEL/CEIL(C) mg/m³	OSHA PELs TWA ppm	TWA mg/m³	STEL/CEIL(C) ppm	STEL/CEIL(C) mg/m³	NIOSH RELs TWA ppm	TWA mg/m³	STEL/CEIL(C) ppm	STEL/CEIL(C) mg/m³	DFG MAKs TWA ppm	TWA mg/m³	PEAK/CEIL(C) ppm	PEAK/CEIL(C) mg/m³	AIHA WEELs TWA ppm	TWA mg/m³	STEL/CEIL(C) ppm	STEL/CEIL(C) mg/m³	CARCINOGENICITY CATEGORY
1,5-Naphthalenediamine 2243-62-1													Skin; Sh								IARC-3 MAK-2
1,5-Naphthalene diisocyanate (NDI) 3173-72-6									0.005	0.04	C 0.02*	C 0.17* *10-min	Sa								IARC-3 MAK-3B
1,8-Naphthalic anhydride 81-84-5													Sh								
Naphthenate, Na-, Ca-, K- 61790-13-4; 61789-36-4; 66072-08-0																					MAK-3B
Naphtho[1,2-b]fluoranthene 111189-32-3																					IARC-3
Naphtho[2,1-a]fluoranthene 203-20-3																					IARC-3
Naphtho[2,3-e]pyrene 193-09-9																					IARC-3
α-Naphthylamine (1-Naphthylamine) 134-32-7					See 29 CFR 1910.1003				See Pocket Guide App. A												IARC-3 NIOSH-Ca OSHA-Ca
β-Naphthylamine (2-Naphthylamine) 91-59-8		L			See 29 CFR 1910.1003				See Pocket Guide App. A				Skin								IARC-1 OSHA-Ca MAK-1 TLV-A1 NIOSH-Ca NTP-K

SUBSTANCE / CAS#	ACGIH® TLVs® TWA ppm	ACGIH® TLVs® TWA mg/m³	ACGIH® TLVs® STEL/CEIL(C) ppm	ACGIH® TLVs® STEL/CEIL(C) mg/m³	OSHA PELs TWA ppm	OSHA PELs TWA mg/m³	OSHA PELs STEL/CEIL(C) ppm	OSHA PELs STEL/CEIL(C) mg/m³	NIOSH RELs TWA ppm	NIOSH RELs TWA mg/m³	NIOSH RELs STEL/CEIL(C) ppm	NIOSH RELs STEL/CEIL(C) mg/m³	DFG MAKs TWA ppm	DFG MAKs TWA mg/m³	DFG MAKs PEAK/CEIL(C) ppm	DFG MAKs PEAK/CEIL(C) mg/m³	AIHA WEELs TWA ppm	AIHA WEELs TWA mg/m³	AIHA WEELs STEL/CEIL(C) ppm	AIHA WEELs STEL/CEIL(C) mg/m³	CARCINOGENICITY CATEGORY
Natural gas 8006-14-2	Refer to Appendix F: Minimal Oxygen Content																				
Natural rubber latex, as inhalable allergenic proteins 9003-31-0; 9006-04-6	0.0001 I													Sah							
Nemalite, fibrous dust 1317-43-7																					MAK-3B
Neon 7440-01-9	NIC-withdraw TLV®; refer to Appendix F: Minimal Oxygen Content (Simple asphyxiant (D))																				
NIAX® Catalyst ESN (Dimethylaminopropionitrile/ bis[2-dimethylamino]ethyl ether mixture) 62765-93-9										minimize exposure *See* Pocket Guide App. C											
Nickel, alloys														for Nickel alloys containing bio-available Nickel, *see* Nickel and Nickel compounds							IARC-2B
Nickel [7440-02-0] **compounds**										0.015* *as Ni				There is sufficient evidence of sensitizing effects on the respiratory tract only for water-soluble Nickel compounds Inhalable fraction Sah							IARC-1 MAK-1 NIOSH-Ca NTP-K

Skin; (SEN) NIC-DSEN; RSEN

See Pocket Guide App. A

SUBSTANCE CAS#	ACGIH® TLVs® TWA ppm	ACGIH® TLVs® TWA mg/m³	ACGIH® TLVs® STEL/CEIL(C) ppm	ACGIH® TLVs® STEL/CEIL(C) mg/m³	OSHA PELs TWA ppm	OSHA PELs TWA mg/m³	OSHA PELs STEL/CEIL(C) ppm	OSHA PELs STEL/CEIL(C) mg/m³	NIOSH RELs TWA ppm	NIOSH RELs TWA mg/m³	NIOSH RELs STEL/CEIL(C) ppm	NIOSH RELs STEL/CEIL(C) mg/m³	DFG MAKs TWA ppm	DFG MAKs TWA mg/m³	DFG MAKs PEAK/CEIL(C) ppm	DFG MAKs PEAK/CEIL(C) mg/m³	AIHA WEELs TWA ppm	AIHA WEELs TWA mg/m³	AIHA WEELs STEL/CEIL(C) ppm	AIHA WEELs STEL/CEIL(C) mg/m³	CARCINOGENICITY CATEGORY
Nickel, elemental 7440-02-0		1.5 I				1				0.015* *as Ni See Pocket Guide App. A				There is sufficient evidence of sensitizing effects on the respiratory tract only for water-soluble Nickel compounds Inhalable fraction Sah							IARC-2B MAK-1 NTP-K TLV-A5
Nickel, insoluble compounds, as Ni 7440-02-0		0.2 I* *Inorganic only				1				0.015* *as Ni See Pocket Guide App. A											NIOSH-Ca NTP-K TLV-A1
Nickel, soluble compounds, as Ni 7440-02-0		0.1 I* *Inorganic only				1				0.015* *as Ni See Pocket Guide App. A											NIOSH-Ca NTP-K TLV-A4
Nickel acetate 373-02-4										0.015* *as Ni See Pocket Guide App. A				and similar soluble salts Inhalable fraction Sah							MAK-1 NIOSH-Ca NTP-K
Nickel carbonate 3333-67-3										0.015* *as Ni See Pocket Guide App. A				Inhalable fraction Sah							IARC-1 MAK-1 NIOSH-Ca NTP-K
Nickel carbonyl, as Ni 13463-39-3	(0.05)	(0.12)	NIC-C 0.05	NIC-C 0.35 NIC-A3	0.001	0.007			0.001	0.007 See Pocket Guide App. A											EPA-B2 IARC-1 NIOSH-Ca NTP-K
Nickel chloride 7718-54-9		See Nickel, soluble compounds, as Ni				1* *as Ni				0.015* *as Ni See Pocket Guide App. A				Inhalable fraction Sah							IARC-1 MAK-1 NIOSH-Ca NTP-K
Nickel dioxide 12035-36-8										0.015* *as Ni See Pocket Guide App. A				Inhalable fraction Sah							IARC-1 MAK-1 NIOSH-Ca NTP-K

SUBSTANCE CAS#	ACGIH® TLVs® TWA ppm	ACGIH® TLVs® TWA mg/m³	ACGIH® TLVs® STEL/CEIL(C) ppm	ACGIH® TLVs® STEL/CEIL(C) mg/m³	OSHA PELs TWA ppm	OSHA PELs TWA mg/m³	OSHA PELs STEL/CEIL(C) ppm	OSHA PELs STEL/CEIL(C) mg/m³	NIOSH RELs TWA ppm	NIOSH RELs TWA mg/m³	NIOSH RELs STEL/CEIL(C) ppm	NIOSH RELs STEL/CEIL(C) mg/m³	DFG MAKs TWA ppm	DFG MAKs TWA mg/m³	DFG MAKs PEAK/CEIL(C) ppm	DFG MAKs PEAK/CEIL(C) mg/m³	AIHA WEELs TWA ppm	AIHA WEELs TWA mg/m³	AIHA WEELs STEL/CEIL(C) ppm	AIHA WEELs STEL/CEIL(C) mg/m³	CARCINOGENICITY CATEGORY
Nickel hydroxide 12054-48-7										0.015* *as Ni See Pocket Guide App. A				Inhalable fraction Sah							IARC-1 MAK-1 NIOSH-Ca NTP-K
Nickel oxide 1313-99-1		See Nickel, insoluble compounds, as Ni				1* *as Ni				0.015* *as Ni See Pocket Guide App. A				Inhalable fraction Sah							IARC-1 MAK-1 NIOSH-Ca NTP-K
Nickel refinery dust																					EPA-A
Nickel sesquioxide 1314-06-3		See Nickel, insoluble compounds, as Ni				1* *as Ni				0.015* *as Ni See Pocket Guide App. A				Inhalable fraction Sah							IARC-1 MAK-1 NIOSH-Ca NTP-K
Nickel subsulfide 12035-72-2		See Nickel, soluble compounds, as Ni								0.015* *as Ni See Pocket Guide App. A				Inhalable fraction Sah							EPA-A NTP-K IARC-1 MAK-1 NIOSH-Ca
Nickel sulfate 7786-81-4		See Nickel, soluble compounds, as Ni				1* *as Ni				0.015* *as Ni See Pocket Guide App. A				Inhalable fraction Sah							IARC-1 MAK-1 NIOSH-Ca NTP-K
Nickel sulfide 16812-54-7														Inhalable fraction Sah							IARC-1 MAK-1 NTP-K
Nicotine 54-11-5	0.5				0.5				0.5					Skin							
	Skin				Skin				Skin												
Nifurthiazole (2-[2-Form-ylhydrazino]-4-[5-nitro-2-furyl]thiazole) 3570-75-0																					IARC-2B

SUBSTANCE / CAS#	ACGIH® TLVs® TWA ppm	TWA mg/m³	STEL/CEIL(C) ppm	mg/m³	OSHA PELs TWA ppm	TWA mg/m³	STEL/CEIL(C) ppm	mg/m³	NIOSH RELs TWA ppm	TWA mg/m³	STEL/CEIL(C) ppm	mg/m³	DFG MAKs TWA ppm	TWA mg/m³	PEAK/CEIL(C) ppm	mg/m³	AIHA WEELs TWA ppm	TWA mg/m³	STEL/CEIL(C) ppm	mg/m³	CARCINOGENICITY CATEGORY
Niridazole 61-57-4																					IARC-2B
Nithiazide 139-94-6																					IARC-3
Nitrapyrin (2-Chloro-6-(trichloromethyl) pyridine) 1929-82-4		10		20	15*; 5**				10*; 5**		20*										TLV-A4
					*Total dust **Respirable fraction				*Total dust **Respirable fraction												
Nitric acid 7697-37-2	2	5.2	4	10	2	5			2	5	4	10									
Nitric oxide 10102-43-9	25	31			25	30			25	30			0.5	0.63	I (2)						
		BEI$_M$											D								
Nitrilotriacetic acid 139-13-9													avoid simultaneous exposure to Iron compounds								IARC-2B* MAK-3A** NTP-R *and its salts **and its sodium salts
5-Nitroacenaphthene 602-87-9																					IARC-2B MAK-2
4-Nitro-4'-aminodi-phenylamine-2-sulfonic acid 91-29-2													Sh								
2-Nitro-4-aminophenol (4-Amino-2-nitrophenol) 119-34-6													Skin								IARC-3 MAK-3B

SUBSTANCE / CAS#	ACGIH® TLVs® TWA ppm	ACGIH® TLVs® TWA mg/m³	ACGIH® TLVs® STEL/CEIL(C) ppm	ACGIH® TLVs® STEL/CEIL(C) mg/m³	OSHA PELs TWA ppm	OSHA PELs TWA mg/m³	OSHA PELs STEL/CEIL(C) ppm	OSHA PELs STEL/CEIL(C) mg/m³	NIOSH RELs TWA ppm	NIOSH RELs TWA mg/m³	NIOSH RELs STEL/CEIL(C) ppm	NIOSH RELs STEL/CEIL(C) mg/m³	DFG MAKs TWA ppm	DFG MAKs TWA mg/m³	DFG MAKs PEAK/CEIL(C) ppm	DFG MAKs PEAK/CEIL(C) mg/m³	AIHA WEELs TWA ppm	AIHA WEELs TWA mg/m³	AIHA WEELs STEL/CEIL(C) ppm	AIHA WEELs STEL/CEIL(C) mg/m³	CARCINOGENICITY CATEGORY
Nitroaniline, p-isomer 100-01-6		3 Skin; BEI$_M$			1 Skin	6			3 Skin				Skin								MAK-3A TLV-A4
5-Nitro-o-anisidine 99-59-2																					IARC-3
2-Nitroanisole 91-23-6																					IARC-2B MAK-2 NTP-R
9-Nitroanthracene 602-60-8																					IARC-3
7-Nitrobenz[a]anthracene 20268-51-3																					IARC-3
3-Nitrobenzanthrone 17117-34-9																					IARC-2B
Nitrobenzene 98-95-3	1 Skin; BEI	5			1 Skin	5			1 Skin	5			Skin								EPA-L NTP-R IARC-2B TLV-A3 MAK-3B
6-Nitrobenzo[a]pyrene 63041-90-7																					IARC-3

SUBSTANCE / CAS#	ACGIH® TLVs® TWA ppm	mg/m³	STEL/CEIL(C) ppm	mg/m³	OSHA PELs TWA ppm	mg/m³	STEL/CEIL(C) ppm	mg/m³	NIOSH RELs TWA ppm	mg/m³	STEL/CEIL(C) ppm	mg/m³	DFG MAKs TWA ppm	mg/m³	PEAK/CEIL(C) ppm	mg/m³	AIHA WEELs TWA ppm	mg/m³	STEL/CEIL(C) ppm	mg/m³	CARCINOGENICITY CATEGORY
4-(2-Nitrobutyl)mor-pholine (70% w/v) [2224-44-4] **and 4,4′-(2-Ethyl-2-nitro-1,3-pro-panediyl)bismorpho-line (20% w/v)** [1854-23-5] **mixture**													0.5	4.2	I (2)						
													Sh; D								
Nitrochlorobenzene, m-isomer (1-Chloronitro-benzene) 121-73-3													Skin								IARC-3
Nitrochlorobenzene, o-isomer (2-Chloronitro-benzene) 88-73-3													Skin								IARC-3 MAK-3B
Nitrochlorobenzene, p-isomer (4-Chloronitro-benzene) 100-00-5	0.1	0.64			1						Skin See Pocket Guide App. A		Skin								IARC-3 MAK-3B NIOSH-Ca TLV-A3
	Skin; BEI_M				Skin																
6-Nitrochrysene 7496-02-8																					IARC-2A NTP-R
Nitrocumene, p-isomer 1817-47-6													Sh								
4-Nitrodiphenyl (4-Nitrobiphenyl) 92-93-3	Skin; L				See 29 CFR 1910.1003				See Pocket Guide App. A				Skin								IARC-3 TLV-A2 MAK-2 NIOSH-Ca OSHA-Ca
Nitroethane 79-24-3	100	307			100	310			100	310			100	310	II (4)						
													D								

SUBSTANCE / CAS#	ACGIH® TLVs® TWA ppm	ACGIH® TLVs® TWA mg/m³	ACGIH® TLVs® STEL/CEIL(C) ppm	ACGIH® TLVs® STEL/CEIL(C) mg/m³	OSHA PELs TWA ppm	OSHA PELs TWA mg/m³	OSHA PELs STEL/CEIL(C) ppm	OSHA PELs STEL/CEIL(C) mg/m³	NIOSH RELs TWA ppm	NIOSH RELs TWA mg/m³	NIOSH RELs STEL/CEIL(C) ppm	NIOSH RELs STEL/CEIL(C) mg/m³	DFG MAKs TWA ppm	DFG MAKs TWA mg/m³	DFG MAKs PEAK/CEIL(C) ppm	DFG MAKs PEAK/CEIL(C) mg/m³	AIHA WEELs TWA ppm	AIHA WEELs TWA mg/m³	AIHA WEELs STEL/CEIL(C) ppm	AIHA WEELs STEL/CEIL(C) mg/m³	CARCINOGENICITY CATEGORY
Nitrofen 1836-75-5																					IARC-2B* NTP-R *technical grade
3-Nitrofluoranthene 892-21-7																					IARC-3
2-Nitrofluorene 607-57-8																					IARC-2B
Nitrofural (Nitrofurazone) 59-87-0																					IARC-3
Nitrofurantoin 67-20-9																					IARC-3
1-[(5-Nitrofurfurylidene) amino]-2-imidazolidi- none 555-84-0																					IARC-2B
Nitrogen 7440-01-9	NIC-withdraw TLV®; refer to Appendix F: Minimal Oxygen Content (Simple asphyxiant(D))																				
Nitrogen dioxide 10102-44-0	0.2	0.38					C 5	C 9			1	1.8	0.5	0.95	I (1) D						MAK-3B TLV-A4
Nitrogen mustard (N-Methyl-bis[2-chloroethyl] amine) 51-75-2											Skin; Sh; 2										IARC-2A MAK-1

SUBSTANCE / CAS#	ACGIH® TLVs® TWA ppm	mg/m³	STEL/CEIL(C) ppm	mg/m³	OSHA PELs TWA ppm	mg/m³	STEL/CEIL(C) ppm	mg/m³	NIOSH RELs TWA ppm	mg/m³	STEL/CEIL(C) ppm	mg/m³	DFG MAKs TWA ppm	mg/m³	PEAK/CEIL(C) ppm	mg/m³	AIHA WEELs TWA ppm	mg/m³	STEL/CEIL(C) ppm	mg/m³	CARCINOGENICITY CATEGORY
Nitrogen mustard hydrochloride (Mechlorethamine hydrochloride) 55-86-7																					NTP-R
Nitrogen mustard N-oxide 126-85-2																					IARC-2B
Nitrogen trifluoride 7783-54-2	10	29			10	29			10	29											BEI$_M$
Nitroglycerin (NG) 55-63-0	0.05	0.46					C 0.2	C 2		0.1			0.01	0.094	II (1)						MAK-3B
		Skin				Skin				Skin				Skin; C							
Nitroguanidine 556-88-7																					EPA-D
Nitromethane 75-52-5	20	50			100	250															IARC-2B MAK-3B NTP-R TLV-A3
														Skin							
1-Nitronaphthalene 86-57-7																					IARC-3 MAK-3B
2-Nitronaphthalene 581-89-5						See Pocket Guide App. A															IARC-3 NIOSH-Ca* MAK-2 *since metabolized to β-Naphthylamine
2-Nitro-p-phenylenediamine (1,4-Diamino-2-nitrobenzene) 5307-14-2														Skin; Sh							IARC-3 MAK-3B

SUBSTANCE / CAS#	ACGIH® TLVs® TWA ppm	ACGIH® TLVs® TWA mg/m³	ACGIH® TLVs® STEL/CEIL(C) ppm	ACGIH® TLVs® STEL/CEIL(C) mg/m³	OSHA PELs TWA ppm	OSHA PELs TWA mg/m³	OSHA PELs STEL/CEIL(C) ppm	OSHA PELs STEL/CEIL(C) mg/m³	NIOSH RELs TWA ppm	NIOSH RELs TWA mg/m³	NIOSH RELs STEL/CEIL(C) ppm	NIOSH RELs STEL/CEIL(C) mg/m³	DFG MAKs TWA ppm	DFG MAKs TWA mg/m³	DFG MAKs PEAK/CEIL(C) ppm	DFG MAKs PEAK/CEIL(C) mg/m³	AIHA WEELs TWA ppm	AIHA WEELs TWA mg/m³	AIHA WEELs STEL/CEIL(C) ppm	AIHA WEELs STEL/CEIL(C) mg/m³	CARCINOGENICITY CATEGORY
3-Nitroperylene 20589-63-3																					IARC-3
1-Nitropropane 108-03-2	25	91			25	90			25	90			25	92	I (4)						TLV-A4
													See 2-Nitropropane when measurably contaminated with that isomer D								
2-Nitropropane 79-46-9	10	36			25	90			*See* Pocket Guide App. A						Skin						IARC-2B NTP-R MAK-2 TLV-A3 NIOSH-Ca
Nitropyrenes 789-07-1; 5522-43-0; 28767-61-5; 57835-92-4; 63021-86-3; 75321-19-6; 78432-19-6																					IARC-2A*; 2B**, 3*** MAK-3B**** NTP-R* *1-Nitropyrene **4-Nitropyrene ***2-Nitropyrene ****mono-, di-, tri-, tetra- isomers
N'-Nitrosoanaba-sine (NAB) 37620-20-5																					IARC-3
N'-Nitrosoanata-bine (NAT) 71267-22-6																					IARC-3
N-Nitrosodi-n-butyl-amine (DBN) 924-16-3											Skin										EPA-B2 IARC-2B MAK-2 NTP-R
N-Nitrosodiethanolamine (NDELA) 1116-54-7											Skin										EPA-B2 IARC-2B MAK-2 NTP-R

SUBSTANCE / CAS#	ACGIH® TLVs® TWA ppm	mg/m³	STEL/CEIL(C) ppm	mg/m³	OSHA PELs TWA ppm	mg/m³	STEL/CEIL(C) ppm	mg/m³	NIOSH RELs TWA ppm	mg/m³	STEL/CEIL(C) ppm	mg/m³	DFG MAKs TWA ppm	mg/m³	PEAK/CEIL(C) ppm	mg/m³	AIHA WEELs TWA ppm	mg/m³	STEL/CEIL(C) ppm	mg/m³	CARCINOGENICITY CATEGORY
N-Nitrosodiethylamine (NDEA) 55-18-5													Skin								EPA-B2 IARC-2A MAK-2 NTP-R
N-Nitrosodiisopropyl-amine 601-77-4													Skin								MAK-2
N-Nitrosodimethylamine (N,N-Dimethylnitrosoamine) 62-75-9	Skin; L				*See* 29 CFR 1910.1003				*See* Pocket Guide App. A				Skin								EPA-B2 NTP-R IARC-2A OSHA-Ca MAK-2 TLV-A3 NIOSH-Ca
N-Nitrosodiphenyl-amine 86-30-6																					EPA-B2 IARC-3 MAK-3B
p-Nitrosodiphenyl-amine 156-10-5																					IARC-3
N-Nitrosodi-n-propyl-amine (NDPA) 621-64-7													Skin								EPA-B2 IARC-2B MAK-2 NTP-R
N-Nitrosoethylphenyl-amine 612-64-6													Skin								MAK-2
N-Nitroso-N-ethylurea 759-73-9																					IARC-2A NTP-R
N-Nitrosofolic acid 29291-35-8																					IARC-3

SUBSTANCE CAS#	ACGIH® TLVs® TWA ppm	mg/m³	STEL/CEIL(C) ppm	mg/m³	OSHA PELs TWA ppm	mg/m³	STEL/CEIL(C) ppm	mg/m³	NIOSH RELs TWA ppm	mg/m³	STEL/CEIL(C) ppm	mg/m³	DFG MAKs TWA ppm	mg/m³	PEAK/CEIL(C) ppm	mg/m³	AIHA WEELs TWA ppm	mg/m³	STEL/CEIL(C) ppm	mg/m³	CARCINOGENICITY CATEGORY
N-Nitrosoguvacine 55557-01-2																					IARC-3
N-Nitrosoguvacoline 55557-02-3																					IARC-3
N-Nitrosohydroxy-proline 30310-80-6																					IARC-3
3-(N-Nitrosomethyl-amino)propion-aldehyde 85502-23-4																					IARC-3
4-(N-Nitrosomethyl-amino)-4-(3-pyridyl)-1-butanal (NNA) 64091-90-3																					IARC-3
4-(N-Nitrosomethyl-amino)-1-(3-pyridyl)-1-butanone 64091-91-4																					IARC-1 NTP-R
N-Nitrosomethylethyl-amine 10595-95-6														Skin							EPA-B2 IARC-2B MAK-2
N-Nitrosomethyl-phenylamine 614-00-6														Skin							MAK-2
N-Nitroso-N-methylurea 684-93-5																					IARC-2A NTP-R

SUBSTANCE / CAS#	ACGIH® TLVs® TWA ppm	mg/m³	STEL/CEIL(C) ppm	mg/m³	OSHA PELs TWA ppm	mg/m³	STEL/CEIL(C) ppm	mg/m³	NIOSH RELs TWA ppm	mg/m³	STEL/CEIL(C) ppm	mg/m³	DFG MAKs TWA ppm	mg/m³	PEAK/CEIL(C) ppm	mg/m³	AIHA WEELs TWA ppm	mg/m³	STEL/CEIL(C) ppm	mg/m³	CARCINOGENICITY CATEGORY
N-Nitrosomethylvinyl-amine 4549-40-0																					IARC-2B NTP-R
N-Nitrosomorpholine (NMOR) 59-89-2															Skin						IARC-2B MAK-2 NTP-R
N′-Nitrosonornicotine (NNN) 16543-55-8																					IARC-1 NTP-R
N-Nitrosopiperidine (NPIP) 100-75-4															Skin						IARC-2B MAK-2 NTP-R
N-Nitrosoproline 7519-36-0																					IARC-3
N-Nitrosopyrrolidine (NPYR) 930-55-2															Skin						EPA-B2 IARC-2B MAK-2 NTP-R
N-Nitrososarcosine 13256-22-9																					IARC-2B NTP-R
Nitrotoluene, m-isomer (3-Nitrotoluene) 99-08-1	2	11			5	30			2	11			Skin								IARC-3 MAK-3B
	Skin; BEI_M				Skin				Skin												
Nitrotoluene, o-isomer (2-Nitrotoluene) 88-72-2	2	11			5	30			2	11			Skin; 3B								IARC-2A MAK-2 NTP-R
	Skin; BEI_M				Skin				Skin												

SUBSTANCE / CAS#	ACGIH® TLVs® TWA ppm	mg/m³	STEL/CEIL(C) ppm	mg/m³	OSHA PELs TWA ppm	mg/m³	STEL/CEIL(C) ppm	mg/m³	NIOSH RELs TWA ppm	mg/m³	STEL/CEIL(C) ppm	mg/m³	DFG MAKs TWA ppm	mg/m³	PEAK/CEIL(C) ppm	mg/m³	AIHA WEELs TWA ppm	mg/m³	STEL/CEIL(C) ppm	mg/m³	CARCINOGENICITY CATEGORY
Nitrotoluene, p-isomer (4-Nitrotoluene) 99-99-0	2	11			5	30			2	11											IARC-3 MAK-3B
	Skin; BEI$_M$				Skin				Skin				Skin								
5-Nitro-o-toluidine (4-Nitro-2-aminotoluene) 99-55-8	1 I																				IARC-3 MAK-2 TLV-A3
Nitrous oxide 10024-97-2	50	90							25*	46*			100	180	II (2)						TLV-A4
									*over the time exposed; for exposure to waste anesthetic gases						C						
Nitrovin 804-36-4																					IARC-3
Nodularins 118399-22-7																					IARC-3
Nonane 111-84-2	200	1050							200	1050											
Nonane, all isomers 111-84-2; 3522-94-9	TLV® withdrawn; *see* Nonane																				
Nonabromodiphenyl ether 63936-56-1																					EPA-D
n-Nonyl mercaptan 1455-21-6											C 0.5*	C 3.3*									
										*15-min										

SUBSTANCE CAS#	ACGIH® TLVs® TWA ppm	ACGIH® TLVs® TWA mg/m³	ACGIH® TLVs® STEL/CEIL(C) ppm	ACGIH® TLVs® STEL/CEIL(C) mg/m³	OSHA PELs TWA ppm	OSHA PELs TWA mg/m³	OSHA PELs STEL/CEIL(C) ppm	OSHA PELs STEL/CEIL(C) mg/m³	NIOSH RELs TWA ppm	NIOSH RELs TWA mg/m³	NIOSH RELs STEL/CEIL(C) ppm	NIOSH RELs STEL/CEIL(C) mg/m³	DFG MAKs TWA ppm	DFG MAKs TWA mg/m³	DFG MAKs PEAK/CEIL(C) ppm	DFG MAKs PEAK/CEIL(C) mg/m³	AIHA WEELs TWA ppm	AIHA WEELs TWA mg/m³	AIHA WEELs STEL/CEIL(C) ppm	AIHA WEELs STEL/CEIL(C) mg/m³	CARCINOGENICITY CATEGORY
Norethisterone 68-22-4																					NTP-R
Nuisance particles						*See* Particles not otherwise classified/regulated								*See* Dust, general threshold limit value							
Nylon 6 25038-54-4																					IARC-3
Oakmoss extracts														Sh							
Ochratoxin A 303-47-9														3B							IARC-2B MAK-2 NTP-R
Octabromodiphenyl ether 32536-52-0																					EPA-D
Octachloronaphthalene 2234-13-1	0.1		0.3	Skin	0.1		Skin		0.1		0.3	Skin									
Octadecyl mercaptan 2885-00-9									C 0.5*		C 5.9*	*15-min									
Octane, all isomers 111-65-9; 540-84-1	300	1401			500	2350		n-Octane only	75	350	C 385*	C 1800* *15-min CAS: 111-65-9 only	500	2400	II (2) except Trimethylpentane isomers D						EPA-II* *CAS: 540-84-1 (oral)

SUBSTANCE CAS#	ACGIH® TLVs® TWA ppm	ACGIH® TLVs® TWA mg/m³	ACGIH® TLVs® STEL/CEIL(C) ppm	ACGIH® TLVs® STEL/CEIL(C) mg/m³	OSHA PELs TWA ppm	OSHA PELs TWA mg/m³	OSHA PELs STEL/CEIL(C) ppm	OSHA PELs STEL/CEIL(C) mg/m³	NIOSH RELs TWA ppm	NIOSH RELs TWA mg/m³	NIOSH RELs STEL/CEIL(C) ppm	NIOSH RELs STEL/CEIL(C) mg/m³	DFG MAKs TWA ppm	DFG MAKs TWA mg/m³	DFG MAKs PEAK/CEIL(C) ppm	DFG MAKs PEAK/CEIL(C) mg/m³	AIHA WEELs TWA ppm	AIHA WEELs TWA mg/m³	AIHA WEELs STEL/CEIL(C) ppm	AIHA WEELs STEL/CEIL(C) mg/m³	CARCINOGENICITY CATEGORY
1-Octanol 111-87-5																	50				
1-Octene 111-66-0																	75				
Octogen 2691-41-0																					EPA-D
2-Octyl-4-isothiazolin-3-one 26530-20-1													0.05 I		I (2)						
													Skin; Sh; C								
n-Octyl mercaptan 111-88-6												C 0.5*	C 3*								
												*15-min									
Oil mist, mineral 8012-95-1		5				5			5		10										
	TLV® withdrawn; *see* Mineral oil																				
Oil Orange SS 2646-17-5																					IARC-2B
Olaquindox 23696-28-8																					MAK-3B
													SP; 2							
Oleic acid 112-80-1																					MAK-3A

| SUBSTANCE | ACGIH® TLVs® | | | | OSHA PELs | | | | NIOSH RELs | | | | DFG MAKs | | | | AIHA WEELs | | | | CARCINOGENICITY |
| | TWA | | STEL/CEIL(C) | | TWA | | STEL/CEIL(C) | | TWA | | STEL/CEIL(C) | | TWA | | PEAK/CEIL(C) | | TWA | | STEL/CEIL(C) | | CATEGORY |
CAS#	ppm	mg/m³	ppm	mg/m³	ppm	mg/m³	ppm	mg/m³	ppm	mg/m³	ppm	mg/m³	ppm	mg/m³	ppm	mg/m³	ppm	mg/m³	ppm	mg/m³	
Orange I 523-44-4																					IARC-3
Orange G 1936-15-8																					IARC-3
Oryzalin 19044-88-3																					EPA-C
Osmium tetroxide 20816-12-0	0.0002	0.0016	0.0006	0.0047		0.002*			0.0002	0.002	0.0006	0.006									
					*as Os																
Oxalic acid 144-62-7		1		2		1				1		2									
Oxazepam 604-75-1																					IARC-2B
p,p'-Oxybis(benzene- sulfonyl hydrazide) 80-51-3		0.1 I																			
Oxygen difluoride 7783-41-7			C 0.05	C 0.11	0.05	0.1					C 0.05	C 0.1									
Oxymetholone 434-07-1																					NTP-R

SUBSTANCE / CAS#	ACGIH® TLVs® TWA ppm	mg/m³	STEL/CEIL(C) ppm	mg/m³	OSHA PELs TWA ppm	mg/m³	STEL/CEIL(C) ppm	mg/m³	NIOSH RELs TWA ppm	mg/m³	STEL/CEIL(C) ppm	mg/m³	DFG MAKs TWA ppm	mg/m³	PEAK/CEIL(C) ppm	mg/m³	AIHA WEELs TWA ppm	mg/m³	STEL/CEIL(C) ppm	mg/m³	CARCINOGENICITY CATEGORY
Oxyphenbutazone 129-20-4																					IARC-3
Ozone [10028-15-6] Heavy work Moderate work Light work Light, moderate, or heavy workload	0.05 0.08 0.1 0.2	0.1 0.16 0.2 0.4 ≤ 2 hours			0.1	0.2					C 0.1	C 0.2									MAK-3B TLV-A4
Palladium chloride [7647-10-1] **and other bio-available Pd(II) compounds**														Sh							
Papain 9001-73-4														Sa							
Paraffin wax fume 8002-74-2		2								2											
Paraquat 4685-14-7		0.5 0.1 **R** as the cation				0.5* *Respirable dust Skin															
Paraquat dichloride 1910-42-5						0.5* *Respirable dust Skin				0.1* *Respirable dust Skin			0.1 **I** Skin		I (1)						EPA-C
Paraquat methosulfate 2074-50-2						0.5* *Respirable dust Skin															

SUBSTANCE CAS#	ACGIH® TLVs® TWA ppm	TWA mg/m³	STEL/CEIL(C) ppm	mg/m³	OSHA PELs TWA ppm	mg/m³	STEL/CEIL(C) ppm	mg/m³	NIOSH RELs TWA ppm	mg/m³	STEL/CEIL(C) ppm	mg/m³	DFG MAKs TWA ppm	mg/m³	PEAK/CEIL(C) ppm	mg/m³	AIHA WEELs TWA ppm	mg/m³	STEL/CEIL(C) ppm	mg/m³	CARCINOGENICITY CATEGORY
Parasorbic acid 10048-32-5																					IARC-3
Parathion 56-38-2	0.05 **IFV** Skin; BEI				0.1 Skin				0.05 Skin				0.1 **I** Skin; D		II (8)						EPA-C IARC-3 TLV-A4
Particles (insoluble or poorly soluble) not otherwise specified	*See* Appendix B in *TLVs® and BEIs®* book																				
Particulates not other-wise classified/regulated (PNOC; PNOR)					15*, 5** or 50 mppcf* 15 mppcf** *Total dust **Respirable fraction								*See* Dust; general threshold limit value								
Patulin 149-29-1																					IARC-3
Penicillic acid 90-65-3																					IARC-3
Pentaborane 19624-22-7	0.005	0.013	0.015	0.039	0.005	0.01			0.005	0.01	0.015	0.03	0.005	0.013	II (2)						
2,2′,4,4′,5-Pentabromo-diphenyl ether (BDE-99) 60348-60-9																					EPA-II
Pentabromodiphenyl ether 32534-81-9																					EPA-D

SUBSTANCE / CAS#	ACGIH® TLVs® TWA ppm	ACGIH® TLVs® TWA mg/m³	ACGIH® TLVs® STEL/CEIL(C) ppm	ACGIH® TLVs® STEL/CEIL(C) mg/m³	OSHA PELs TWA ppm	OSHA PELs TWA mg/m³	OSHA PELs STEL/CEIL(C) ppm	OSHA PELs STEL/CEIL(C) mg/m³	NIOSH RELs TWA ppm	NIOSH RELs TWA mg/m³	NIOSH RELs STEL/CEIL(C) ppm	NIOSH RELs STEL/CEIL(C) mg/m³	DFG MAKs TWA ppm	DFG MAKs TWA mg/m³	DFG MAKs PEAK/CEIL(C) ppm	DFG MAKs PEAK/CEIL(C) mg/m³	AIHA WEELs TWA ppm	AIHA WEELs TWA mg/m³	AIHA WEELs STEL/CEIL(C) ppm	AIHA WEELs STEL/CEIL(C) mg/m³	CARCINOGENICITY CATEGORY
Pentachlorobenzene 608-93-5																					EPA-D
3,4,5,3′,4′-Pentachloro-biphenyl (PCB-126) 57465-28-8																					IARC-1
Pentachlorocyclo-pentadiene 25329-35-5																					EPA-D
2,3,4,7,8-Pentachloro-dibenzofuran 57117-31-4																					IARC-1
Pentachloroethane 76-01-7										handle with caution *See* Pocket Guide App. C			5	42	II (2)						IARC-3
Pentachloronaphthalene 1321-64-8	0.5				0.5				0.5				Skin								IARC-3
	Skin				Skin				Skin												
Pentachloronitro-benzene 82-68-8	0.5																				IARC-3 TLV-A4
Pentachlorophenol 87-86-5	(0.5) NIC-0.5 **IFV** Skin; BEI	NIC-1 **IFV**			0.5 Skin				0.5 Skin				Skin								EPA-L IARC-2B MAK-2 TLV-A3
Pentaerythritol 115-77-5	10				15*; 5** *Total dust **Respirable fraction				10*; 5** *Total dust **Respirable fraction												

SUBSTANCE CAS#	ACGIH® TLVs® TWA ppm	mg/m³	STEL/CEIL(C) ppm	mg/m³	OSHA PELs TWA ppm	mg/m³	STEL/CEIL(C) ppm	mg/m³	NIOSH RELs TWA ppm	mg/m³	STEL/CEIL(C) ppm	mg/m³	DFG MAKs TWA ppm	mg/m³	PEAK/CEIL(C) ppm	mg/m³	AIHA WEELs TWA ppm	mg/m³	STEL/CEIL(C) ppm	mg/m³	CARCINOGENICITY CATEGORY
Pentaerythritol triacrylate 3524-68-3														Sh				1 DSEN			
1,1,1,2,2-Pentafluoro-ethane 354-33-6																	1000				
1,1,1,3,3-Pentafluoro-propane 460-73-1																	300				
Pentane, all isomers 78-78-4; 109-66-0; 463-82-1	(600) NIC-1000	(1770) NIC-2950			1000	2950			120	350 CAS: 109-66-0 only	C 610*	C 1800* *15-min	1000	3000	II (2) C						
2,4-Pentanedione 123-54-6	25	102 Skin											20	83 Skin; C	II (2)						
Pentanol, all isomers 71-41-0; 75-84-3; 75-85-4; 123-51-3; 137-32-6; 584-02-1; 598-75-4; 6032-29-7; 30899-19-5; 94624-12-1													20	73 C	I (4)		100 CAS: 71-41-0 only				
1-Pentyl acetate (n-Amyl acetate) 628-63-7	50	266	100	532	100	525			100	525			50	270 C	I (1)						
2-Pentyl acetate (sec-Amyl acetate) 626-38-0	50	266	100	532	125	650			125	650			50	270 D	I (1)						

SUBSTANCE / CAS#	ACGIH® TLVs® TWA ppm	TWA mg/m³	STEL/CEIL(C) ppm	STEL/CEIL(C) mg/m³	OSHA PELs TWA ppm	TWA mg/m³	STEL/CEIL(C) ppm	STEL/CEIL(C) mg/m³	NIOSH RELs TWA ppm	TWA mg/m³	STEL/CEIL(C) ppm	STEL/CEIL(C) mg/m³	DFG MAKs TWA ppm	TWA mg/m³	PEAK/CEIL(C) ppm	PEAK/CEIL(C) mg/m³	AIHA WEELs TWA ppm	TWA mg/m³	STEL/CEIL(C) ppm	STEL/CEIL(C) mg/m³	CARCINOGENICITY CATEGORY
3-Pentyl acetate 620-11-1	50	266	100	532									50	270	I (1) D						
4-Pentyl acetate (tert-Amyl-acetate) 625-16-1	50	226	100	532									50	270	I (1) D						
Pentyl mercaptan 110-66-7											C 0.5* *15-min	C 2.1*									
Pepsin 9001-75-6														Sa							
Peracetic acid 79-21-0			NIC-0.4* *IFV	NIC-1.24* NIC-A4																	MAK-3B
Perchlorate and perchlorate salts 7601-89-0; 7778-74-7; 7790-98-9; 7791-03-9																					EPA-NL
Perchloromethyl mercaptan 594-42-3	0.1	0.76			0.1	0.8			0.1	0.8											
Perchloryl fluoride 7616-94-6	3	13	6	25	3	13.5			3	14	6	28									
Perfluorobutyl ethylene (PFBE) 19430-93-4	100	1023																			

SUBSTANCE / CAS#	ACGIH® TLVs® TWA ppm	mg/m³	STEL/CEIL(C) ppm	mg/m³	OSHA PELs TWA ppm	mg/m³	STEL/CEIL(C) ppm	mg/m³	NIOSH RELs TWA ppm	mg/m³	STEL/CEIL(C) ppm	mg/m³	DFG MAKs TWA ppm	mg/m³	PEAK/CEIL(C) ppm	mg/m³	AIHA WEELs TWA ppm	mg/m³	STEL/CEIL(C) ppm	mg/m³	CARCINOGENICITY CATEGORY
Perfluoroisobutylene 382-21-8			C 0.01	C 0.082																	
Perfluorooctanesulfonic acid (PFOS) **and its salts** 1763-23-1													0.01 **I**		II (8) Skin; B						MAK-3B
Perfluorooctanoic acid and its inorganic salts 335-67-1													0.005 **I**		II (8) Skin; B						MAK-4
Perlite 93763-70-3	TLV® withdrawn due to insufficient data				15*; 5** *Total dust **Respirable fraction				10*; 5** *Total dust **Respirable fraction												
Permethrin 52645-53-1																					IARC-3
Persulfates, as persulfate 7727-21-1; 7727-27-1		0.1																			
Perylene 198-55-0																					IARC-3
Petasitenine 60102-37-6																					IARC-3
Petroleum distillates, hydrotreated light 64742-47-8	20	140													II (2) C						MAK-3B

SUBSTANCE / CAS#	ACGIH® TLVs® TWA ppm	TWA mg/m³	STEL/CEIL(C) ppm	mg/m³	OSHA PELs TWA ppm	TWA mg/m³	STEL/CEIL(C) ppm	mg/m³	NIOSH RELs TWA ppm	TWA mg/m³	STEL/CEIL(C) ppm	mg/m³	DFG MAKs TWA ppm	TWA mg/m³	PEAK/CEIL(C) ppm	mg/m³	AIHA WEELs TWA ppm	TWA mg/m³	STEL/CEIL(C) ppm	mg/m³	CARCINOGENICITY CATEGORY
Petroleum distillates, Naphtha (Rubber solvent) 8002-05-9	Rubber solvent TLV® withdrawn				500	2000			350		C 1800* *15-min										IARC-3
Phenacetin 62-44-2																					IARC-1 NTP-R
Phenanthrene 85-01-8														Skin							EPA-D IARC-3
Phenazopyridine hydrochloride 136-40-3																					IARC-2B NTP-R
Phenelzine sulfate 156-51-4																					IARC-3
Phenicarbazide 103-03-7																					IARC-3
Phenol 108-95-2	5	19		Skin; BEI	5	19		Skin	5	19	C 15.6* C 60* *15-min	Skin				Skin; 3B					EPA-I; D IARC-3 MAK-3B TLV-A4
Phenolphthalein 77-09-8																					IARC-2B NTP-R
Phenothiazine 92-84-2		5		Skin						5		Skin									

SUBSTANCE / CAS#	ACGIH® TLVs® TWA ppm	TWA mg/m³	STEL/CEIL(C) ppm	mg/m³	OSHA PELs TWA ppm	mg/m³	STEL/CEIL(C) ppm	mg/m³	NIOSH RELs TWA ppm	mg/m³	STEL/CEIL(C) ppm	mg/m³	DFG MAKs TWA ppm	mg/m³	PEAK/CEIL(C) ppm	mg/m³	AIHA WEELs TWA ppm	mg/m³	STEL/CEIL(C) ppm	mg/m³	CARCINOGENICITY CATEGORY
Phenoxybenzamine hydrochloride 63-92-3																					IARC-2B NTP-R
2-Phenoxyethanol (Ethylene glycol mono- phenyl ether) 122-99-6													20	110	I (2)						Skin; C
Phenylbutazone 50-33-9																					IARC-3
Phenylenediamine, m-isomer 108-45-2		0.1																			IARC-3 MAK-3B TLV-A4 Skin; Sh
Phenylenediamine, o-isomer 95-54-5		0.1																			MAK-3B TLV-A3 Sh
Phenylenediamine, p-isomer 106-50-3		0.1				0.1				0.1				0.1 I	II (2)						IARC-3 MAK-3B TLV-A4 Skin (OSHA) Skin (NIOSH) Skin; Sh; C
2-Phenyl-1-ethanol 60-12-8																					Skin
Phenyl ether, vapor 101-84-8	1	7	2	14	1	7			1	7			1	7.1	I (1)						C
Phenyl ether/biphenyl mixture, vapor 8004-13-5					1	7			1	7											

SUBSTANCE / CAS#	ACGIH® TLVs® TWA ppm	mg/m³	STEL/CEIL(C) ppm	mg/m³	OSHA PELs TWA ppm	mg/m³	STEL/CEIL(C) ppm	mg/m³	NIOSH RELs TWA ppm	mg/m³	STEL/CEIL(C) ppm	mg/m³	DFG MAKs TWA ppm	mg/m³	PEAK/CEIL(C) ppm	mg/m³	AIHA WEELs TWA ppm	mg/m³	STEL/CEIL(C) ppm	mg/m³	CARCINOGENICITY CATEGORY
Phenyl glycidyl ether (PGE) 122-60-1	0.1	0.6			10	60					C 1* *15-min See Pocket Guide App. A	C 6*									IARC-2B MAK-2 NIOSH-Ca TLV-A3
	Skin; (SEN) NIC-DSEN												Skin; Sh								
Phenylhydrazine 100-63-0	0.1	0.44			5	22					C 0.14* Skin *120-min See Pocket Guide App. A	C 0.6*									MAK-3B NIOSH-Ca TLV-A3
		Skin				Skin							Skin; Sh								
Phenyl isocyanate 103-71-9	NIC-0.005	NIC-0.024	NIC-0.02	NIC-0.1											Sah						
		NIC-DSEN; RSEN																			
Phenyl mercaptan 108-98-5	0.1	0.45									C 0.1* *15-min	C 0.5*									
		Skin																			
N-Phenyl-1-naph-thylamine 90-30-2														Sh							
N-Phenyl-β-naph-thylamine 135-88-6		L									See Pocket Guide App. A			Sh							IARC-3 NIOSH-Ca* MAK-3B TLV-A4 *since metabolized to β-Naphthylamine
Phenylphenol, o-isomer 90-43-7																					IARC-3
Phenylphosphine 638-21-1			C 0.05	C 0.23							C 0.05	C 0.25									
Phenyltin compounds													0.0004*	0.002 I		II (2)					MAK-4
													*can also be found as vapor Skin; C							

SUBSTANCE / CAS#	ACGIH® TLVs® TWA ppm	TWA mg/m³	STEL/CEIL(C) ppm	STEL/CEIL(C) mg/m³	OSHA PELs TWA ppm	TWA mg/m³	STEL/CEIL(C) ppm	STEL/CEIL(C) mg/m³	NIOSH RELs TWA ppm	TWA mg/m³	STEL/CEIL(C) ppm	STEL/CEIL(C) mg/m³	DFG MAKs TWA ppm	TWA mg/m³	PEAK/CEIL(C) ppm	PEAK/CEIL(C) mg/m³	AIHA WEELs TWA ppm	TWA mg/m³	STEL/CEIL(C) ppm	STEL/CEIL(C) mg/m³	CARCINOGENICITY CATEGORY
Phenytoin 57-41-0																					IARC-2B NTP-R
Phorate 298-02-2		0.05 **IFV** Skin; BEI_A								0.05 Skin		0.2									TLV-A4
Phosgene (Carbonyl chloride) 75-44-5	0.1	0.4			0.1	0.4			0.1	0.4	C 0.2* *15-min	C 0.8*	0.1	0.41	I (2) C						EPA-II
Phosphine 7803-51-2	0.3	0.42	1	1.4	0.3	0.4			0.3	0.4	1	1	0.1	0.14	II (2) C						EPA-D
2-Phosphono-1,2-4-butanetricarboxylic acid 37971-36-1																		10 (H)			
Phosphoric acid 7664-38-2		1		3		1				1		3		2 I	I (2) C						
Phosphorus-32, as phosphate 14596-37-3																					IARC-1
Phosphorus, White 7723-14-0										0.1				0.01 I	II (2) C						EPA-D
Phosphorus, Yellow 12185-10-3	0.02	0.1				0.1				0.1				0.01 I	II (2) C						

SUBSTANCE CAS#	ACGIH® TLVs® TWA ppm	mg/m³	STEL/CEIL(C) ppm	mg/m³	OSHA PELs TWA ppm	mg/m³	STEL/CEIL(C) ppm	mg/m³	NIOSH RELs TWA ppm	mg/m³	STEL/CEIL(C) ppm	mg/m³	DFG MAKs TWA ppm	mg/m³	PEAK/CEIL(C) ppm	mg/m³	AIHA WEELs TWA ppm	mg/m³	STEL/CEIL(C) ppm	mg/m³	CARCINOGENICITY CATEGORY
Phosphorus oxy-chloride 10025-87-3	0.1	0.63							0.1	0.6	0.5	3	0.2	1.3	I (1) C						
Phosphorus penta-chloride 10026-13-8	0.1	0.85				1				1				1 I	I (1) C						
Phosphorus penta-sulfide 1314-80-3		1		3		1				1		3									
Phosphorus pentoxide 1314-56-3														2 I	I (2) C						
Phosphorus trichloride 7719-12-2	0.2	1.1	0.5	2.8	0.5	3			0.2	1.5	0.5	3	0.5	2.8	I (1) C						
Phthalic acid, m-isomer (Isophthalate) 121-91-5														5 I	I (2) C		10* 5 R *Total dust				
Phthalic anhydride 85-44-9	1	6.1 (SEN) NIC-DSEN; RSEN			2	12			1	6				Sa							TLV-A4
Phthalodinitrile, m-isomer 626-17-5	5 IFV									5											
Phthalodinitrile, o-isomer 91-15-6	1 IFV																				

SUBSTANCE / CAS#	ACGIH® TLVs® TWA ppm	TWA mg/m³	STEL/CEIL(C) ppm	STEL/CEIL(C) mg/m³	OSHA PELs TWA ppm	TWA mg/m³	STEL/CEIL(C) ppm	STEL/CEIL(C) mg/m³	NIOSH RELs TWA ppm	TWA mg/m³	STEL/CEIL(C) ppm	STEL/CEIL(C) mg/m³	DFG MAKs TWA ppm	TWA mg/m³	PEAK/CEIL(C) ppm	PEAK/CEIL(C) mg/m³	AIHA WEELs TWA ppm	TWA mg/m³	STEL/CEIL(C) ppm	STEL/CEIL(C) mg/m³	CARCINOGENICITY CATEGORY
Phytases													Sa								
Picene 213-46-7																					IARC-3
Picloram 1918-02-1	10				15*; 5**																IARC-3 TLV-A4
					*Total dust **Respirable fraction																
2-Picoline 109-06-8																	2		5		
																	Skin				
3-Picoline 108-99-6																	2		5		
																	Skin				
4-Picoline 108-89-4																	2		5		
																	Skin				
Picric acid (2,4,6-Trinitrophenol) 88-89-1	0.1				0.1				0.1			0.3									MAK-3B
					Skin				Skin				Skin; Sh								
Picryl chloride 88-88-0																					
												Sh								
Pindone (2-Pivalyl-1,3-indandione) 83-26-1	0.1				0.1				0.1												

SUBSTANCE / CAS#	ACGIH® TLVs® TWA ppm	mg/m³	STEL/CEIL(C) ppm	mg/m³	OSHA PELs TWA ppm	mg/m³	STEL/CEIL(C) ppm	mg/m³	NIOSH RELs TWA ppm	mg/m³	STEL/CEIL(C) ppm	mg/m³	DFG MAKs TWA ppm	mg/m³	PEAK/CEIL(C) ppm	mg/m³	AIHA WEELs TWA ppm	mg/m³	STEL/CEIL(C) ppm	mg/m³	CARCINOGENICITY CATEGORY
Piperazine and salts, as Piperazine 110-85-0	0.03 **IFV**	0.1 **IFV**																			TLV-A4
	(SEN) NIC-DSEN; RSEN												CAS: 110-85-0 only Sah								
Piperazine dihydro-chloride 142-64-3	TLV® withdrawn; *see* Piperazine and salts, as Piperazine								5												
Piperidine 110-89-4																	1				
															Skin						
Piperonyl butoxide 51-03-6																					IARC-3
Plaster of Paris (Calcium sulfate hemihydrate) 26499-65-0					15*; 5**				10*; 5**												
					*Total dust **Respirable fraction				*Total dust **Respirable fraction												
Platinum, metal 7440-06-4	1								1												
Platinum, soluble salts, as Pt 7440-06-4	0.002				0.002				0.002						C 0.002						
													Chloroplatinates Sah								
Plutonium 7440-07-5																					IARC-1
Polyacrylic acid 9003-01-4																					IARC-3

SUBSTANCE CAS#	ACGIH® TLVs® TWA ppm	ACGIH® TLVs® TWA mg/m³	ACGIH® TLVs® STEL/CEIL(C) ppm	ACGIH® TLVs® STEL/CEIL(C) mg/m³	OSHA PELs TWA ppm	OSHA PELs TWA mg/m³	OSHA PELs STEL/CEIL(C) ppm	OSHA PELs STEL/CEIL(C) mg/m³	NIOSH RELs TWA ppm	NIOSH RELs TWA mg/m³	NIOSH RELs STEL/CEIL(C) ppm	NIOSH RELs STEL/CEIL(C) mg/m³	DFG MAKs TWA ppm	DFG MAKs TWA mg/m³	DFG MAKs PEAK/CEIL(C) ppm	DFG MAKs PEAK/CEIL(C) mg/m³	AIHA WEELs TWA ppm	AIHA WEELs TWA mg/m³	AIHA WEELs STEL/CEIL(C) ppm	AIHA WEELs STEL/CEIL(C) mg/m³	CARCINOGENICITY CATEGORY
Polyalphaolefins														5 R C	II (4)						
Polybrominated biphenyls (PBBs) 59536-65-1																					IARC-2B NTP-R
Polychlorinated biphenyls (PCBs) 1336-36-3																					EPA-B2 IARC-2A NIOSH-Ca NTP-R
Polychlorinated dibenzo-p-dioxins, excluding 2,3,7,8-tetrachlorodibenzo-p-dioxin																					IARC-3
Polychlorinated dibenzofurans 136677-10-6																					IARC-3
Polychlorophenols and their sodium salts, mixed exposures																					IARC-2B
Polychloroprene 9010-98-4																					IARC-3
Polyethylene 9002-88-4																					IARC-3

SUBSTANCE CAS#	ACGIH® TLVs® TWA ppm	ACGIH® TLVs® TWA mg/m³	ACGIH® TLVs® STEL/CEIL(C) ppm	ACGIH® TLVs® STEL/CEIL(C) mg/m³	OSHA PELs TWA ppm	OSHA PELs TWA mg/m³	OSHA PELs STEL/CEIL(C) ppm	OSHA PELs STEL/CEIL(C) mg/m³	NIOSH RELs TWA ppm	NIOSH RELs TWA mg/m³	NIOSH RELs STEL/CEIL(C) ppm	NIOSH RELs STEL/CEIL(C) mg/m³	DFG MAKs TWA ppm	DFG MAKs TWA mg/m³	DFG MAKs PEAK/CEIL(C) ppm	DFG MAKs PEAK/CEIL(C) mg/m³	AIHA WEELs TWA ppm	AIHA WEELs TWA mg/m³	AIHA WEELs STEL/CEIL(C) ppm	AIHA WEELs STEL/CEIL(C) mg/m³	CARCINOGENICITY CATEGORY
Polyethylene glycol (average molecular weight 200-600)														1000 I due to possible mist formation, exposure should be minimized C		II (8)		10 (H); MW > 200 CAS: 25322-68-3			
Polymethylene poly-phenyl isocyanate (Polymeric MDI) 9016-87-9														0.05 I Skin; Sah; C		I (1)					EPA-CBD; D IARC-3 MAK-4
Polymethyl methacry-late 9011-14-7																					IARC-3
Polypropylene 9003-07-0																					IARC-3
Polypropylene glycol(s) 25322-69-4																		10 (H)			IARC-3
Polystyrene 9003-53-6																					IARC-3
Polytetrafluoro-ethylene 9002-84-0																					IARC-3
Polyurethane foams 9009-54-5																					IARC-3
Polyvinyl acetate 9003-20-7																					IARC-3

Substance / CAS#	ACGIH® TLVs® TWA ppm	TWA mg/m³	STEL/CEIL(C) ppm	STEL/CEIL(C) mg/m³	OSHA PELs TWA ppm	TWA mg/m³	STEL/CEIL(C) ppm	STEL/CEIL(C) mg/m³	NIOSH RELs TWA ppm	TWA mg/m³	STEL/CEIL(C) ppm	STEL/CEIL(C) mg/m³	DFG MAKs TWA ppm	TWA mg/m³	PEAK/CEIL(C) ppm	PEAK/CEIL(C) mg/m³	AIHA WEELs TWA ppm	TWA mg/m³	STEL/CEIL(C) ppm	STEL/CEIL(C) mg/m³	Carcinogenicity Category
Polyvinyl alcohol 9002-89-5																					IARC-3
Polyvinyl chloride (PVC) 9002-86-2	1 R												1.5 R 4 I C								IARC-3 TLV-A4
Polyvinyl pyrrolidone 9003-39-8																					IARC-3
Ponceau MX 3761-53-3																					IARC-2B
Ponceau 3R 3564-09-8																					IARC-2B
Ponceau SX 4548-53-2																					IARC-3
Portland cement 65997-15-1	1 R E				50 mppcf or 15*; 5** *Total dust **Respirable fraction				10*; 5** *Total dust **Respirable fraction				Dust* *Quartz and chromate fractions must be evaluated as such (valid only for low-chromate cement containing < 2 ppm of Cr (VI). Refer to the Cr (VI) cmpds for cement with a higher Cr (VI) content)								MAK-3B TLV-A4
Potassium bis(2-hydroxy-ethyl)dithiocarbamate 23746-34-1																					IARC-3

SUBSTANCE / CAS#	ACGIH® TLVs® TWA ppm	TWA mg/m³	STEL/CEIL(C) ppm	STEL/CEIL(C) mg/m³	OSHA PELs TWA ppm	TWA mg/m³	STEL/CEIL(C) ppm	STEL/CEIL(C) mg/m³	NIOSH RELs TWA ppm	TWA mg/m³	STEL/CEIL(C) ppm	STEL/CEIL(C) mg/m³	DFG MAKs TWA ppm	TWA mg/m³	PEAK/CEIL(C) ppm	PEAK/CEIL(C) mg/m³	AIHA WEELs TWA ppm	TWA mg/m³	STEL/CEIL(C) ppm	STEL/CEIL(C) mg/m³	CARCINOGENICITY CATEGORY
Potassium bromate 7758-01-2																		0.1			IARC-2B
Potassium cyanide, as CN 151-50-8	*See* Hydrogen cyanide and cyanide salts, as CN				*See* Cyanides						C 4.7*	C 5* *10-min	5.0 I		II (1) Skin; C						
Potassium hydroxide 1310-58-3				C 2								C 2									
Potassium titanates, fibrous dust																					MAK-2
Prazepam 2955-38-6																					IARC-3
Prednimustine 29069-24-7																					IARC-3
Prednisone 53-03-2																					IARC-3
Printing inks																					IARC-3
Procarbazine hydrochloride 366-70-1																					IARC-2A NTP-R

SUBSTANCE / CAS#	ACGIH® TLVs® TWA ppm	mg/m³	STEL/CEIL(C) ppm	mg/m³	OSHA PELs TWA ppm	mg/m³	STEL/CEIL(C) ppm	mg/m³	NIOSH RELs TWA ppm	mg/m³	STEL/CEIL(C) ppm	mg/m³	DFG MAKs TWA ppm	mg/m³	PEAK/CEIL(C) ppm	mg/m³	AIHA WEELs TWA ppm	mg/m³	STEL/CEIL(C) ppm	mg/m³	CARCINOGENICITY CATEGORY
Prochloraz 67747-09-5																					EPA-C
Proflavine salts																					IARC-3
Pronetalol hydro-chloride 51-02-5																					IARC-3
Propane 74-98-6	Refer to Appendix F: Minimal Oxygen Content				1000	1800			1000	1800			1000	1800 D	II (4)						
Propane sultone (1,3-Propane sultone) 1120-71-4	L								See Pocket Guide App. A				Skin								IARC-2B TLV-A3 MAK-2 NIOSH-Ca NTP-R
n-Propanol (n-Propyl alcohol) 71-23-8	100	246			200	500			200	500	250	625									TLV-A4
									Skin												
2-Propanol (Isopropanol; Isopropyl alcohol) 67-63-0	200	492	400	984	400	980			400	980	500	1225	200	500	II (2)						IARC-3 TLV-A4
	BEI												C								
Propargyl alcohol 107-19-7	1	2.3							1	2			2	4.7	I (2)						
	Skin								Skin				Skin; D								
Propargyl bromide 106-96-7																	0.1				
																	Skin			

SUBSTANCE / CAS#	ACGIH® TLVs® TWA ppm	TWA mg/m³	STEL/CEIL(C) ppm	STEL/CEIL(C) mg/m³	OSHA PELs TWA ppm	TWA mg/m³	STEL/CEIL(C) ppm	STEL/CEIL(C) mg/m³	NIOSH RELs TWA ppm	TWA mg/m³	STEL/CEIL(C) ppm	STEL/CEIL(C) mg/m³	DFG MAKs TWA ppm	TWA mg/m³	PEAK/CEIL(C) ppm	PEAK/CEIL(C) mg/m³	AIHA WEELs TWA ppm	TWA mg/m³	STEL/CEIL(C) ppm	STEL/CEIL(C) mg/m³	CARCINOGENICITY CATEGORY
Propham 122-42-9																					IARC-3
β-Propiolactone 57-57-8	0.5	1.5			*See* 29 CFR 1910.1003				*See* Pocket Guide App. A				Skin								IARC-2B OSHA-Ca MAK-2 TLV-A3 NIOSH-Ca NTP-R
Propionaldehyde 123-38-6	20	48															20				EPA-II
Propionic acid 79-09-4	10	30							10	30	15	45	10	31	I (2)						
														C							
Propionitrile 107-12-0									6	14											
Propoxur 114-26-1		0.5							0.5					2 I	II (8)						TLV-A3
		BEI_A																			
2-Propoxyethanol (Ethylene glycol mono-n-propyl ether) 2807-30-9													20	86	I (2)						
												Skin; C									
2-Propoxyethyl acetate (Ethylene glycol monopropyl ether acetate) 20706-25-6													20	120	I (2)						
												Skin; C									
n-Propyl acetate 109-60-4	200	835	250	1040	200	840			200	840	250	1050	100	420	I (2)						
												D									

SUBSTANCE CAS#	ACGIH® TLVs® TWA ppm	mg/m³	STEL/CEIL(C) ppm	mg/m³	OSHA PELs TWA ppm	mg/m³	STEL/CEIL(C) ppm	mg/m³	NIOSH RELs TWA ppm	mg/m³	STEL/CEIL(C) ppm	mg/m³	DFG MAKs TWA ppm	mg/m³	PEAK/CEIL(C) ppm	mg/m³	AIHA WEELs TWA ppm	mg/m³	STEL/CEIL(C) ppm	mg/m³	CARCINOGENICITY CATEGORY
n-Propyl carbamate 627-12-3																					IARC-3
Propylene 115-07-1	500	860																			IARC-3 TLV-A4
Propylene dichloride (1,2-Dichloropropane) 78-87-5	10	46 (SEN) NIC-DSEN			75	350			*See* Pocket Guide App. A												IARC-3 MAK-3B NIOSH-Ca TLV-A4
Propylene glycol 57-55-6																	10				
Propylene glycol dinitrate (PGDN) 6423-43-4	0.05	0.34 Skin; BEI_M							0.05 Skin	0.3			0.05 Skin	0.34	II (1)						
Propylene oxide (1,2-Epoxypropane) 75-56-9	2	4.8 (SEN) NIC-DSEN			100	240			*See* Pocket Guide App. A				2 Sh; C	4.8	I (2)						EPA-B2 NTP-R IARC-2B TLV-A3 MAK-4 NIOSH-Ca
Propyleneimine (2-Methylaziridine) 75-55-8	0.2 Skin	0.5	0.4	1	2 Skin	5			2 Skin *See* Pocket Guide App. A	5			Skin; 3B								IARC-2B TLV-A3 MAK-2 NIOSH-Ca NTP-R
n-Propyl mercaptan 107-03-9											C 0.5* *15-min	C 1.6*									
n-Propyl nitrate 627-13-4	25	107 BEI_M	40	172	25	110			25	105	40	170									

SUBSTANCE / CAS#	ACGIH® TLVs® TWA ppm	ACGIH® TLVs® TWA mg/m³	ACGIH® TLVs® STEL/CEIL(C) ppm	ACGIH® TLVs® STEL/CEIL(C) mg/m³	OSHA PELs TWA ppm	OSHA PELs TWA mg/m³	OSHA PELs STEL/CEIL(C) ppm	OSHA PELs STEL/CEIL(C) mg/m³	NIOSH RELs TWA ppm	NIOSH RELs TWA mg/m³	NIOSH RELs STEL/CEIL(C) ppm	NIOSH RELs STEL/CEIL(C) mg/m³	DFG MAKs TWA ppm	DFG MAKs TWA mg/m³	DFG MAKs PEAK/CEIL(C) ppm	DFG MAKs PEAK/CEIL(C) mg/m³	AIHA WEELs TWA ppm	AIHA WEELs TWA mg/m³	AIHA WEELs STEL/CEIL(C) ppm	AIHA WEELs STEL/CEIL(C) mg/m³	CARCINOGENICITY CATEGORY
Propylthiouracil 51-52-5																					IARC-2B NTP-R
Ptaquiloside 87625-62-5																					IARC-3
Pyrene 129-00-0														Skin							EPA-D IARC-3
Pyrethrum 8003-34-7		5				5				5			does not apply for the constituents of insecticides or synthetic derivatives Sh								TLV-A4
Pyridine 110-86-1	1	3.1			5	15			5	15			Skin								IARC-3 MAK-3B TLV-A3
Pyrido[3,4-c]psoralen 85878-62-2																					IARC-3
Pyrimethamine 58-14-0																					IARC-3
Pyrrolidine 123-75-1														Skin							
Quercetin 117-39-5																					IARC-3

SUBSTANCE / CAS#	ACGIH® TLVs® TWA ppm	mg/m³	STEL/CEIL(C) ppm	mg/m³	OSHA PELs TWA ppm	mg/m³	STEL/CEIL(C) ppm	mg/m³	NIOSH RELs TWA ppm	mg/m³	STEL/CEIL(C) ppm	mg/m³	DFG MAKs TWA ppm	mg/m³	PEAK/CEIL(C) ppm	mg/m³	AIHA WEELs TWA ppm	mg/m³	STEL/CEIL(C) ppm	mg/m³	CARCINOGENICITY CATEGORY
Quinoline 91-22-5																	0.001	Skin			EPA-L; B2
Quinone (p-Benzoquinone) 106-51-4	0.1	0.44			0.1	0.4			0.1	0.4			Sh; 3B								IARC-3 MAK-3B
Reserpine 50-55-5																					IARC-3 NTP-R
Resorcinol 108-46-3	10	45	20	90					10	45	20	90	Sh								IARC-3 TLV-A4
Retrorsine 480-54-6																					IARC-3
Rhodamine B 81-88-9																					IARC-3
Rhodamine 6G 989-38-8																					IARC-3
Rhodium, elemental 7440-16-6		1				0.1				0.1											MAK-3B TLV-A4
Rhodium, insoluble compounds, as Rh		1				0.1				0.1											MAK-3B* TLV-A4 *inorganic only

SUBSTANCE CAS#	ACGIH® TLVs® TWA ppm	ACGIH® TLVs® TWA mg/m³	ACGIH® TLVs® STEL/CEIL(C) ppm	ACGIH® TLVs® STEL/CEIL(C) mg/m³	OSHA PELs TWA ppm	OSHA PELs TWA mg/m³	OSHA PELs STEL/CEIL(C) ppm	OSHA PELs STEL/CEIL(C) mg/m³	NIOSH RELs TWA ppm	NIOSH RELs TWA mg/m³	NIOSH RELs STEL/CEIL(C) ppm	NIOSH RELs STEL/CEIL(C) mg/m³	DFG MAKs TWA ppm	DFG MAKs TWA mg/m³	DFG MAKs PEAK/CEIL(C) ppm	DFG MAKs PEAK/CEIL(C) mg/m³	AIHA WEELs TWA ppm	AIHA WEELs TWA mg/m³	AIHA WEELs STEL/CEIL(C) ppm	AIHA WEELs STEL/CEIL(C) mg/m³	CARCINOGENICITY CATEGORY
Rhodium, soluble compounds, as Rh	0.01				0.001				0.001												MAK-3B* TLV-A4 *inorganic only
Ricinus protein															Sa						
Riddelliine 23246-96-0																					NTP-R
Rifampicin 13292-46-1																					IARC-3
Ripazepam 26308-28-1																					IARC-3
Ronnel 299-84-3		5 IFV				15				10											TLV-A4
		BEI$_A$																			
Rosin core solder thermal decomposition products (colophony) 8050-09-7	(SEN); L; NIC-DSEN; RSEN														Sh						
Rosin core solder, pyrolysis products, as formaldehyde	See Rosin core solder thermal decomposition products								0.1												NIOSH-Ca* *in presence of Formaldehyde, Acetaldehyde or Malon aldehyde
									See Pocket Guide Apps. A and C												
Rotenone, commercial 83-79-4	5				5				5						Skin						TLV-A4

SUBSTANCE / CAS#	ACGIH® TLVs® TWA ppm	mg/m³	STEL/CEIL(C) ppm	mg/m³	OSHA PELs TWA ppm	mg/m³	STEL/CEIL(C) ppm	mg/m³	NIOSH RELs TWA ppm	mg/m³	STEL/CEIL(C) ppm	mg/m³	DFG MAKs TWA ppm	mg/m³	PEAK/CEIL(C) ppm	mg/m³	AIHA WEELs TWA ppm	mg/m³	STEL/CEIL(C) ppm	mg/m³	CARCINOGENICITY CATEGORY
Rouge	TLV® withdrawn; *see* Iron oxide				15*; 5**																
	*Total dust **Respirable fraction																				
Rubber components													Sh								
Rugulosin 23537-16-8																					IARC-3
Saccharated iron oxide 8047-67-4																					IARC-3
Saccharin [81-07-2] and its salts																					IARC-3
Safrole 94-59-7																					IARC-2B NTP-R
Scarlet Red 85-83-6																					IARC-3
Selenious acid 7783-00-8																					EPA-D
Selenium [7782-49-2] compounds, as Se	0.2				0.2				0.2												EPA-D IARC-3

SUBSTANCE / CAS#	ACGIH® TLVs® TWA ppm	ACGIH® TLVs® TWA mg/m³	ACGIH® TLVs® STEL/CEIL(C) ppm	ACGIH® TLVs® STEL/CEIL(C) mg/m³	OSHA PELs TWA ppm	OSHA PELs TWA mg/m³	OSHA PELs STEL/CEIL(C) ppm	OSHA PELs STEL/CEIL(C) mg/m³	NIOSH RELs TWA ppm	NIOSH RELs TWA mg/m³	NIOSH RELs STEL/CEIL(C) ppm	NIOSH RELs STEL/CEIL(C) mg/m³	DFG MAKs TWA ppm	DFG MAKs TWA mg/m³	DFG MAKs PEAK/CEIL(C) ppm	DFG MAKs PEAK/CEIL(C) mg/m³	AIHA WEELs TWA ppm	AIHA WEELs TWA mg/m³	AIHA WEELs STEL/CEIL(C) ppm	AIHA WEELs STEL/CEIL(C) mg/m³	CARCINOGENICITY CATEGORY
Selenium [7782-49-2], inorganic compounds, as Se														0.02 I	II (8)						MAK-3B
													Skin; C								
Selenium, metal 7782-49-2		0.2								0.2* *except Selenium hexafluoride				0.02 I Skin; C	II (8)						EPA-D IARC-3 MAK-3B
Selenium hexa-fluoride, as Se 7783-79-1	0.05	0.4			0.05	0.4			0.05												IARC-3
Selenium sulfide 7446-34-6		0.2* *as Se				0.2* *as Se				0.2* *as Se				0.02 I Skin; C	II (8)						EPA-B2 IARC-3 MAK-3B NTP-R
Semicarbazide hydro-chloride 563-41-7																					IARC-3
Seneciphylline 480-81-9																					IARC-3
Senkirkine 2318-18-5																					IARC-3
Sepiolite, fibrous dust e.g., 15501-74-3; 18307-23-8																					IARC-3 MAK-3B
Sesquiterpene lactone														Sh							

SUBSTANCE / CAS#	ACGIH® TLVs® TWA ppm	TWA mg/m³	STEL/CEIL(C) ppm	STEL/CEIL(C) mg/m³	OSHA PELs TWA ppm	TWA mg/m³	STEL/CEIL(C) ppm	STEL/CEIL(C) mg/m³	NIOSH RELs TWA ppm	TWA mg/m³	STEL/CEIL(C) ppm	STEL/CEIL(C) mg/m³	DFG MAKs TWA ppm	TWA mg/m³	PEAK/CEIL(C) ppm	PEAK/CEIL(C) mg/m³	AIHA WEELs TWA ppm	TWA mg/m³	STEL/CEIL(C) ppm	STEL/CEIL(C) mg/m³	CARCINOGENICITY CATEGORY
Sesone (Sodium-2,4-dichlorophenoxyethyl sulfate) 136-78-7	10				15*; 5** *Total dust **Respirable fraction				10*; 5** *Total dust **Respirable fraction												TLV-A4
Shale oils 68308-34-9																					IARC-1
Shikimic acid 138-59-0																					IARC-3
Sidestream smoke (Passive smoking at the work-place i.e., second-hand smoke)																					IARC-1 MAK-1 NTP-K
Silica, amorphous, diatomaceous earth, calcined 68895-54-9														0.3 R C							IARC-3
Silica, amorphous, diatomaceous earth, uncalcined 61790-53-2	TLV® withdrawn due to insufficient data on single substance exposure				20 mppcf or $\dfrac{80 \text{ mg/m}^3}{\% \text{ SiO}_2}$				6 *See* Pocket Guide App. C					4 I C							IARC-3
Silica, amorphous, precipitated and gel 112926-00-8	TLV® withdrawn due to insufficient data				20 mppcf or $\dfrac{80 \text{ mg/m}^3}{\% \text{ SiO}_2}$				6 *See* Pocket Guide App. C												IARC-3
Silica, amorphous, silica fume 69012-64-2	TLV® withdrawn due to insufficient data																				IARC-3

SUBSTANCE CAS#	ACGIH® TLVs® TWA ppm / mg/m³	STEL/CEIL(C) ppm / mg/m³	OSHA PELs TWA ppm / mg/m³	STEL/CEIL(C) ppm / mg/m³	NIOSH RELs TWA ppm / mg/m³	STEL/CEIL(C) ppm / mg/m³	DFG MAKs TWA ppm / mg/m³	PEAK/CEIL(C) ppm / mg/m³	AIHA WEELs TWA ppm / mg/m³	STEL/CEIL(C) ppm / mg/m³	CARCINOGENICITY CATEGORY
Silica, amorphous, fused 60676-86-0	TLV® withdrawn due to insufficient data		$\dfrac{30\ mg/m^{3}*}{\%\ SiO_2 + 2}$ $\dfrac{250\ mppcf**}{\%\ SiO_2 + 5}$ or $\dfrac{10\ mg/m^{3}**}{\%\ SiO_2 + 2}$ *Total dust **Respirable dust				0.3 **R** including CAS: 7699-41-4 C				IARC-3
Silica, crystalline, cristobalite 14464-46-1	0.025 **R**		1/2 the value calculated from the respirable dust formulae for Quartz		0.05* *Respirable dust See Pocket Guide App. A						IARC-1 NTP-K* MAK-1* TLV-A2 NIOSH-Ca *respirable
Silica, crystalline, α-quartz 14808-60-7	0.025 **R**		$\dfrac{30\ mg/m^{3}*}{\%\ SiO_2 + 2}$ $\dfrac{250\ mppcf**}{\%\ SiO_2 + 5}$ or $\dfrac{10\ mg/m^{3}**}{\%\ SiO_2 + 2}$ *Total dust **Respirable dust		0.05* *Respirable dust See Pocket Guide App. A						IARC-1 MAK-1* NIOSH-Ca NTP-K* TLV-A2 *respirable
Silica, crystalline, tridymite 15468-32-3	TLV® withdrawn due to insufficient data		1/2 the value calculated from the respirable dust formulae for Quartz		0.05* *Respirable dust See Pocket Guide App. A						IARC-1 NIOSH-Ca MAK-1* NTP-K* *respirable
Silica, crystalline, tripoli 1317-95-9	TLV® withdrawn due to insufficient data and unlikely single substance exposure		$\dfrac{30\ mg/m^{3}*}{\%\ SiO_2 + 2}$ $\dfrac{250\ mppcf**}{\%\ SiO_2 + 5}$ or $\dfrac{10\ mg/m^{3}**}{\%\ SiO_2 + 2}$ *Total dust **Respirable dust		0.05* *Respirable dust See Pocket Guide App. A						IARC-1 NIOSH-Ca NTP-K* TLV-A2 *respirable
Silicon 7440-21-3	TLV® withdrawn due to insufficient data		15*; 5** *Total dust **Respirable fraction		10*; 5** *Total dust **Respirable fraction						

SUBSTANCE CAS#	ACGIH® TLVs® TWA ppm	mg/m³	STEL/CEIL(C) ppm	mg/m³	OSHA PELs TWA ppm	mg/m³	STEL/CEIL(C) ppm	mg/m³	NIOSH RELs TWA ppm	mg/m³	STEL/CEIL(C) ppm	mg/m³	DFG MAKs TWA ppm	mg/m³	PEAK/CEIL(C) ppm	mg/m³	AIHA WEELs TWA ppm	mg/m³	STEL/CEIL(C) ppm	mg/m³	CARCINOGENICITY CATEGORY
Silicon carbide, fibrous dust 409-21-2	0.1 f/cc(F) including whiskers				15*; 5** *Total dust **Respirable fraction				10*; 5** *Total dust **Respirable fraction												MAK-2 TLV-A2
Silicon carbide, nonfibrous 409-21-2		10 I 3 R E																			
Silicon tetrahydride (Silane) 7803-62-5	5	6.6			5				5	7											
Silver, metal 7440-22-4		0.1 dust and fume				0.01				0.01				0.1 I D	II (8)						EPA-D
Silver, salts, as Ag														0.01 I D	I (2)						
Silver, soluble compounds, as Ag 7440-22-4		0.01				0.01				0.01											
Simazine 122-34-9	NIC-0.5 I NIC-A4																				IARC-3
Soapstone						20 mppcf*				6*; 3**												

TLV® withdrawn; see Documentation for Talc

*< 1% Crystalline

containing < 1% Quartz

*Total dust **Respirable dust

SUBSTANCE CAS#	ACGIH® TLVs® TWA ppm	mg/m³	STEL/CEIL(C) ppm	mg/m³	OSHA PELs TWA ppm	mg/m³	STEL/CEIL(C) ppm	mg/m³	NIOSH RELs TWA ppm	mg/m³	STEL/CEIL(C) ppm	mg/m³	DFG MAKs TWA ppm	mg/m³	PEAK/CEIL(C) ppm	mg/m³	AIHA WEELs TWA ppm	mg/m³	STEL/CEIL(C) ppm	mg/m³	CARCINOGENICITY CATEGORY
Sodium aluminum fluoride, as F 15096-52-3						2.5				2.5												
Sodium arsenite 7784-46-5	0.01*				0.01*					as As	C 0.002* *15-min See Pocket Guide App. A			as As 3A								EPA-A NTP-K IARC-1 OSHA-Ca MAK-1 TLV-A1 NIOSH-Ca
	*as As				*as As																	
Sodium azide 26628-22-8			C 0.11*	C 0.29**							C 0.1* C 0.3** *as HN₃ **as NaN₃ Skin			0.2 I	D	I (2)						TLV-A4
			*as HN₃ vapor **as NaN₃																			
Sodium bisulfite 7631-90-5		5								5												IARC-3 TLV-A4
Sodium chloroacetate 3926-62-3																			0.5			
Sodium cyanide, as CN 143-33-9	See Hydrogen cyanide and cyanide salts				See Cyanides				applies to other Cyanides, as CN except Hydrogen cyanide		C 4.7* C 5* *10-min			3.8 I Skin; C		II (1)						
Sodium cyclamate 139-05-9																						IARC-3
Sodium diethyldithio-carbamate 148-18-5														2 I Sh; D		II (2)						IARC-3
Sodium fluoroacetate 62-74-8	0.05				0.05				0.05		0.15			0.05 I Skin; B		II (4)						
		Skin				Skin				Skin												

SUBSTANCE / CAS#	ACGIH® TLVs® TWA ppm	mg/m³	STEL/CEIL(C) ppm	mg/m³	OSHA PELs TWA ppm	mg/m³	STEL/CEIL(C) ppm	mg/m³	NIOSH RELs TWA ppm	mg/m³	STEL/CEIL(C) ppm	mg/m³	DFG MAKs TWA ppm	mg/m³	PEAK/CEIL(C) ppm	mg/m³	AIHA WEELs TWA ppm	mg/m³	STEL/CEIL(C) ppm	mg/m³	CARCINOGENICITY CATEGORY
Sodium hydroxide 1310-73-2				C 2		2						C 2									
Sodium hypochlorite 7681-52-9																				2	
Sodium metabisulfite 7681-57-4		5								5											TLV-A4
Sodium persulfate, as S₂O₈ 7775-27-1		0.1																			
														Sah							
Sodium-o-phenyl-phenate 132-27-4																					IARC-2B
Sodium pyrithione 3811-73-2; 15922-78-8														1 I		II (2)					
														Skin; B							
Sodium tetraborate, anhydrous 1330-43-4										1											
	See Borate compounds, inorganic																				
Sodium tetraborate, decahydrate 1303-96-4										5											
	See Borate compounds, inorganic																				
Sodium tetraborate, pentahydrate 12179-04-3										1				5 I		I (1)					
	See Borate compounds, inorganic														C							

S_2O_8

SUBSTANCE CAS#	ACGIH® TLVs® TWA ppm	mg/m³	STEL/CEIL(C) ppm	mg/m³	OSHA PELs TWA ppm	mg/m³	STEL/CEIL(C) ppm	mg/m³	NIOSH RELs TWA ppm	mg/m³	STEL/CEIL(C) ppm	mg/m³	DFG MAKs TWA ppm	mg/m³	PEAK/CEIL(C) ppm	mg/m³	AIHA WEELs TWA ppm	mg/m³	STEL/CEIL(C) ppm	mg/m³	CARCINOGENICITY CATEGORY
Soya bean constituents														Sa							
Spironolactone 52-01-7																					IARC-3
Starch 9005-25-8		10				15*; 5**				10*; 5**											TLV-A4
					*Total dust **Respirable fraction				*Total dust **Respirable dust												
Stearates		10																			TLV-A4
		J																			
Sterigmatocystin 10048-13-2																					IARC-2B
Stoddard solvent 8052-41-3	100	525			500	2900			350		C 1800*										
											*15-min										
Streptozotocin 18883-66-4																					IARC-2B NTP-R
Strontium chromate, as Cr 7789-06-2		0.0005				0.005				0.001 as Cr				as Cr(VI) Skin; Sh; 2							IARC-1 TLV-A2 MAK-1 NIOSH-Ca NTP-K
					See 29 CFR 1910.1026				See Pocket Guide Apps. A and C												
Strychnine 57-24-9		0.15				0.15				0.15											

SUBSTANCE CAS#	ACGIH® TLVs® TWA ppm	ACGIH® TLVs® TWA mg/m³	ACGIH® TLVs® STEL/CEIL(C) ppm	ACGIH® TLVs® STEL/CEIL(C) mg/m³	OSHA PELs TWA ppm	OSHA PELs TWA mg/m³	OSHA PELs STEL/CEIL(C) ppm	OSHA PELs STEL/CEIL(C) mg/m³	NIOSH RELs TWA ppm	NIOSH RELs TWA mg/m³	NIOSH RELs STEL/CEIL(C) ppm	NIOSH RELs STEL/CEIL(C) mg/m³	DFG MAKs TWA ppm	DFG MAKs TWA mg/m³	DFG MAKs PEAK/CEIL(C) ppm	DFG MAKs PEAK/CEIL(C) mg/m³	AIHA WEELs TWA ppm	AIHA WEELs TWA mg/m³	AIHA WEELs STEL/CEIL(C) ppm	AIHA WEELs STEL/CEIL(C) mg/m³	CARCINOGENICITY CATEGORY
Styrene, monomer (Phenylethylene; Vinyl benzene) 100-42-5	20	85 BEI	40	170	100		C 200; 600* *5-min peak in any 3 hrs		50	215	100	425	20	86	II (2) C						IARC-2B MAK-5 NTP-R TLV-A4
Styrene-acrylonitrile copolymers 9003-54-7																					IARC-3
Styrene-butadiene copolymers 9003-55-8																					IARC-3
Styrene-7,8-oxide (1,2-Epoxyethylbenzene) 96-09-3																					IARC-2A NTP-R
Subtilisins 1395-21-7; 9014-01-1		as 100% crystalline active pure enzyme	C 0.00006								0.00006* *60-min				Sa						
Succinic anhydride 108-30-5																					IARC-3
Succinonitrile 110-61-2									6	20											
Sucrose 57-50-1		10			15*; 5** *Total dust **Respirable fraction				10*; 5** *Total dust **Respirable fraction												TLV-A4
Sudan I 842-07-9																					IARC-3

SUBSTANCE / CAS#	ACGIH® TLVs® TWA ppm	mg/m³	STEL/CEIL(C) ppm	mg/m³	OSHA PELs TWA ppm	mg/m³	STEL/CEIL(C) ppm	mg/m³	NIOSH RELs TWA ppm	mg/m³	STEL/CEIL(C) ppm	mg/m³	DFG MAKs TWA ppm	mg/m³	PEAK/CEIL(C) ppm	mg/m³	AIHA WEELs TWA ppm	mg/m³	STEL/CEIL(C) ppm	mg/m³	CARCINOGENICITY CATEGORY
Sudan II 3118-97-6																					IARC-3
Sudan III 85-86-9																					IARC-3
Sudan Brown RR 6416-57-5																					IARC-3
Sudan Red 7B 6368-72-5																					IARC-3
Sulfafurazole (Sulfisoxazole) 127-69-5																					IARC-3
Sulfallate 95-06-7																					IARC-2B NTP-R
Sulfamethazine 57-68-1																					IARC-3
Sulfamethoxazole 723-46-6																					IARC-3
Sulfites																					IARC-3

SUBSTANCE / CAS#	ACGIH® TLVs® TWA ppm	mg/m³	STEL/CEIL(C) ppm	mg/m³	OSHA PELs TWA ppm	mg/m³	STEL/CEIL(C) ppm	mg/m³	NIOSH RELs TWA ppm	mg/m³	STEL/CEIL(C) ppm	mg/m³	DFG MAKs TWA ppm	mg/m³	PEAK/CEIL(C) ppm	mg/m³	AIHA WEELs TWA ppm	mg/m³	STEL/CEIL(C) ppm	mg/m³	CARCINOGENICITY CATEGORY
Sulfometuron methyl 74222-97-2	5																				TLV-A4
Sulfotepp (TEDP) 3689-24-5	0.1 **IFV** Skin; BEI_A				0.2 Skin				0.2 Skin				0.01* *can also be found as vapor Skin; C	0.13 **I**	II (2)						TLV-A4
Sulfur dioxide 7446-09-5		0.25		0.65	5	13			2	5	5	13	1 C	2.7	I (1) C 1	C 2.7					IARC-3 TLV-A4
Sulfur hexafluoride 2551-62-4	1000	5970			1000	6000			1000	6000			1000 D	6100	II (8)						
Sulfuric acid 7664-93-9	0.2 **T**					1				1			0.1 **I** C		I (1) C 0.2						IARC-1* NTP-K* MAK-4 TLV-A2* *refers to Sulfuric acid contained in strong inorganic acid mists
Sulfur monochloride 10025-67-9			C 1	C 5.5	1	6					C 1	C 6									
Sulfur pentafluoride 5714-22-7			C 0.01	C 0.10	0.025	0.25					C 0.01	C 0.1									
Sulfur tetrafluoride 7783-60-0			C 0.1	C 0.44							C 0.1	C 0.4									
Sulfuryl fluoride 2699-79-8	5	21	10	42	5	20			5	20	10	40									

SUBSTANCE / CAS#	ACGIH® TLVs® TWA ppm	ACGIH® TLVs® TWA mg/m³	ACGIH® TLVs® STEL/CEIL(C) ppm	ACGIH® TLVs® STEL/CEIL(C) mg/m³	OSHA PELs TWA ppm	OSHA PELs TWA mg/m³	OSHA PELs STEL/CEIL(C) ppm	OSHA PELs STEL/CEIL(C) mg/m³	NIOSH RELs TWA ppm	NIOSH RELs TWA mg/m³	NIOSH RELs STEL/CEIL(C) ppm	NIOSH RELs STEL/CEIL(C) mg/m³	DFG MAKs TWA ppm	DFG MAKs TWA mg/m³	DFG MAKs PEAK/CEIL(C) ppm	DFG MAKs PEAK/CEIL(C) mg/m³	AIHA WEELs TWA ppm	AIHA WEELs TWA mg/m³	AIHA WEELs STEL/CEIL(C) ppm	AIHA WEELs STEL/CEIL(C) mg/m³	CARCINOGENICITY CATEGORY
Sulprofos 35400-43-2	0.008* *IFV	0.1* Skin; BEI$_A$							1												TLV-A4
Sunset Yellow FCF 2783-94-0																					IARC-3
Symphytine 22571-95-5																					IARC-3
Synthetic vitreous fibers, continuous filament glass fibers	5 I	1 f/cc$^{(F)}$							5* *Total fibrous glass, or 3 f/cc TWA (fib ≤ 3.5 μm diam; ≥ 10 μm length)												IARC-3* TLV-A4 *glass filament
Synthetic vitreous fibers, glass wool fibers		1 f/cc$^{(F)}$							5* *Total fibrous glass, or 3 f/cc TWA (fib ≤ 3.5 μm diam; ≥ 10 μm length)												IARC-3 MAK-2 NTP-R* TLV-A3 *inhalable
Synthetic vitreous fibers, rock wool fibers		1 f/cc$^{(F)}$																			IARC-3 MAK-2 TLV-A3
Synthetic vitreous fibers, slag wool fibers		1 f/cc$^{(F)}$																			IARC-3 MAK-3B TLV-A3
Synthetic vitreous fibers, special purpose glass fibers		1 f/cc$^{(F)}$																			IARC-2B NTP-R* TLV-A3 *inhalable
Synthetic vitreous fibers, refractory ceramic fibers		0.2 f/cc$^{(F)}$																			EPA-B2 IARC-2B MAK-2 TLV-A2

SUBSTANCE / CAS#	ACGIH® TLVs® TWA ppm	mg/m³	STEL/CEIL(C) ppm	mg/m³	OSHA PELs TWA ppm	mg/m³	STEL/CEIL(C) ppm	mg/m³	NIOSH RELs TWA ppm	mg/m³	STEL/CEIL(C) ppm	mg/m³	DFG MAKs TWA ppm	mg/m³	PEAK/CEIL(C) ppm	mg/m³	AIHA WEELs TWA ppm	mg/m³	STEL/CEIL(C) ppm	mg/m³	CARCINOGENICITY CATEGORY
2,4,5-T (2,4,5-Trichloro-phenoxyacetic acid) 93-76-5	10				10				10				2 I		II (2)						TLV-A4
													Skin; C								
Talc, containing no asbestos fibers 14807-96-6	2 R				20 mppcf* *containing < 1% Quartz				2* and < 1% Quartz *Respirable dust												IARC-3 MAK-3B* TLV-A4 *respirable
		E																			
Talc, containing asbestos fibers Use Asbestos TLV–TWA; (K)					Use Asbestos PEL *See* 29 CFR 1910.1001				*See* Asbestos												IARC-1 NTP-K OSHA-Ca TLV-A1
Tall oil, distilled 8002-26-4													Sh* *only applies to Tall oil containing abietic acid								
Tamoxifen 10540-29-1												ˎ									IARC-1 NTP-K
Tannic acid [1401-55-4] **and tannins**																					IARC-3
Tantalum, metal 7440-25-7	TLV® withdrawn due to insufficient data				5				5		10		4 I 1.5 R C								
Tantalum oxide, dusts, as Ta 1314-61-0	TLV® withdrawn due to insufficient data				5				5		10										
Tellurium [13494-80-9] **and compounds, as Te**	0.1* *except Hydrogen telluride				0.1				0.1* *except Tellurium hexafluoride and Bismuth telluride												

SUBSTANCE / CAS#	ACGIH® TLVs® TWA ppm	ACGIH® TLVs® TWA mg/m³	ACGIH® TLVs® STEL/CEIL(C) ppm	ACGIH® TLVs® STEL/CEIL(C) mg/m³	OSHA PELs TWA ppm	OSHA PELs TWA mg/m³	OSHA PELs STEL/CEIL(C) ppm	OSHA PELs STEL/CEIL(C) mg/m³	NIOSH RELs TWA ppm	NIOSH RELs TWA mg/m³	NIOSH RELs STEL/CEIL(C) ppm	NIOSH RELs STEL/CEIL(C) mg/m³	DFG MAKs TWA ppm	DFG MAKs TWA mg/m³	DFG MAKs PEAK/CEIL(C) ppm	DFG MAKs PEAK/CEIL(C) mg/m³	AIHA WEELs TWA ppm	AIHA WEELs TWA mg/m³	AIHA WEELs STEL/CEIL(C) ppm	AIHA WEELs STEL/CEIL(C) mg/m³	CARCINOGENICITY CATEGORY
Tellurium hexafluoride, as Te 7783-80-4	0.02	0.2			0.02	0.2			0.02	0.2											
Temazepam 846-50-4																					IARC-3
Temephos 3383-96-8		1 IFV Skin; BEI$_A$				15*; 5** *Total dust **Respirable fraction				10*; 5** *Total dust **Respirable fraction											TLV-A4
Teniposide 29767-20-2																					IARC-2A
Terbufos 1307-79-9		0.01 IFV Skin; BEI$_A$																			TLV-A4
Terephthalic acid (p-Phthalic acid) 100-21-0		10												5 I C		I (2)					
Terpene polychlorinates 8001-50-1																					IARC-3
Terphenyl, o-, m-, p-isomers 84-15-1; 92-06-8; 92-94-4; 26140-60-3			C 0.53	C 5			C 1	C 9			C 0.5	C 5									
2,2′,4,4′-Tetrabromodiphenyl ether (BDE-47) 5436-43-1																					EPA-II

SUBSTANCE / CAS#	ACGIH® TLVs® TWA ppm	TWA mg/m³	STEL/CEIL(C) ppm	STEL/CEIL(C) mg/m³	OSHA PELs TWA ppm	TWA mg/m³	STEL/CEIL(C) ppm	STEL/CEIL(C) mg/m³	NIOSH RELs TWA ppm	TWA mg/m³	STEL/CEIL(C) ppm	STEL/CEIL(C) mg/m³	DFG MAKs TWA ppm	TWA mg/m³	PEAK/CEIL(C) ppm	PEAK/CEIL(C) mg/m³	AIHA WEELs TWA ppm	TWA mg/m³	STEL/CEIL(C) ppm	STEL/CEIL(C) mg/m³	CARCINOGENICITY CATEGORY
Tetrabromodiphenyl ether 40088-47-9																					EPA-D
1,1,2,2-Tetrabromo-ethane (Acetylene tetrabromide) 79-27-6	0.1 **IFV**	1.4 **IFV**			1	14															
Tetra-n-butyltin compounds													0.004*	0.02 **I**	I (1)						MAK-4
													Skin**; C								
													*can also be found as vapor **for n-butyltin cmpds whose organic ligands are already designated "Sa" or "Sh", these designations also apply								
2,2',5,5'-Tetrachloro-benzidine 15721-02-5																					IARC-3
Tetrachlorocyclopen-tadiene 695-77-2																					EPA-D
2,3,7,8-Tetrachlorodi-benzo-p-dioxin (TCDD) 1746-01-6									*See* Pocket Guide App. A				1•10⁻⁸ **I**		II (8)						IARC-1 MAK-4 NIOSH-Ca NTP-K
													Skin; C								
1,1,1,2-Tetrachloro-2,2-difluoroethane (FC-112a) 76-11-9	100	834			500	4170			500	4170			200	1700	II (2)						
													D								
1,1,2,2-Tetrachloro-1,2-difluoroethane (FC-112) 76-12-0	50	417			500	4170			500	4170			200	1700	II (2)						
													D								

SUBSTANCE / CAS#	ACGIH® TLVs® TWA ppm	mg/m³	STEL/CEIL(C) ppm	mg/m³	OSHA PELs TWA ppm	mg/m³	STEL/CEIL(C) ppm	mg/m³	NIOSH RELs TWA ppm	mg/m³	STEL/CEIL(C) ppm	mg/m³	DFG MAKs TWA ppm	mg/m³	PEAK/CEIL(C) ppm	mg/m³	AIHA WEELs TWA ppm	mg/m³	STEL/CEIL(C) ppm	mg/m³	CARCINOGENICITY CATEGORY
1,1,1,2-Tetrachloro-ethane 630-20-6									handle with caution *See* Pocket Guide App. C												EPA-C IARC-2B
1,1,2,2-Tetrachloro-ethane (Acetylene tetrachloride) 79-34-5	1	6.9		Skin	5	35	Skin		1	7 Skin *See* Pocket Guide Apps. A and C			1	7 Skin; D	II (2)						EPA-L IARC-2B MAK-3B NIOSH-Ca TLV-A3
Tetrachloroethylene (Perchloroethylene) 127-18-4	25	170 BEI	100	685	100		C 200; 300* *5-min peak in any 3 hrs		minimize workplace exposure concentrations *See* Pocket Guide App. A					Skin							EPA-L IARC-2A MAK-3B NIOSH-Ca NTP-R TLV-A3
Tetrachloronaphthalene 1335-88-2		2				2 Skin				2 Skin											
2,3,5,6-Tetrachloro-pyridine 2402-79-1																		5			
Tetrachlorosilane 10026-04-7																			C 1		
Tetrachlorvinphos 22248-79-9																					IARC-3
Tetraethylene glycol diacrylate 17831-71-9										Sh								1 Skin; DSEN			
Tetraethylene glycol dimethacrylate 109-17-1										Sh											

SUBSTANCE / CAS#	ACGIH® TLVs® TWA ppm	mg/m³	STEL/CEIL(C) ppm	mg/m³	OSHA PELs TWA ppm	mg/m³	STEL/CEIL(C) ppm	mg/m³	NIOSH RELs TWA ppm	mg/m³	STEL/CEIL(C) ppm	mg/m³	DFG MAKs TWA ppm	mg/m³	PEAK/CEIL(C) ppm	mg/m³	AIHA WEELs TWA ppm	mg/m³	STEL/CEIL(C) ppm	mg/m³	CARCINOGENICITY CATEGORY
Tetraethylene pentamine 112-57-2																	5				
																	Skin; DSEN				
Tetraethyl lead, as Pb 78-00-2	0.1				0.075				0.075					0.05	II (2)						IARC-3 TLV-A4
	Skin				Skin				Skin				Skin; B								
Tetraethyl pyrophos- phate (TEPP) 107-49-3	0.01 IFV				0.05				0.05				0.005	0.06	II (2)						
	Skin; BEI_A				Skin				Skin				Skin								
1,1,1,2-Tetrafluoroethane (HFC 134a) 811-97-2													1000	4200	II (8)		1000				
														C							
Tetrafluoroethylene (Tetrafluoroethene) 116-14-3	2	8.2																			IARC-2B MAK-2 NTP-R TLV-A3
2,3,3,3-Tetrafluoro- propene 754-12-1																	500				
1,3,3,3-Tetrafluoro- propylene 1645-83-6																	800				
Tetrahydrofuran 109-99-9	50	147	100	295	200	590			200	590	250	735	50	150	I (2)						EPA-S MAK-4 TLV-A3
	Skin												Skin; C								
Tetrahydrofurfuryl alcohol 97-99-4																	0.5				

SUBSTANCE CAS#	ACGIH® TLVs® TWA ppm	mg/m³	STEL/CEIL(C) ppm	mg/m³	OSHA PELs TWA ppm	mg/m³	STEL/CEIL(C) ppm	mg/m³	NIOSH RELs TWA ppm	mg/m³	STEL/CEIL(C) ppm	mg/m³	DFG MAKs TWA ppm	mg/m³	PEAK/CEIL(C) ppm	mg/m³	AIHA WEELs TWA ppm	mg/m³	STEL/CEIL(C) ppm	mg/m³	CARCINOGENICITY CATEGORY
Tetrahydrofurfuryl methacrylate 2455-24-5														Sh							
Tetrahydronaphthalene 119-64-2													2	11	I (1) C						
Tetrahydrothiophene (THT) 110-01-0													50	180	I (1) C						
Tetrakis(hydroxymethyl)-phosphonium chloride 124-64-1		2 (SEN) NIC-DSEN																			IARC-3 TLV-A4
Tetrakis(hydroxymethyl)-phosphonium sulfate 55566-30-8		2 (SEN) NIC-DSEN																			IARC-3 TLV-A4
Tetramethyl lead, as Pb 75-74-1		0.15 Skin				0.075 Skin				0.075 Skin				0.05 Skin; B	II (2)						IARC-3
Tetramethyl succino-nitrile 3333-52-6	0.5	2.8 Skin			0.5	3 Skin			0.5	3 Skin				Skin							
Tetranitromethane 509-14-8	0.005	0.04			1	8			1	8				Skin							IARC-2B MAK-2 NTP-R TLV-A3

SUBSTANCE / CAS#	ACGIH® TLVs® TWA ppm	mg/m³	STEL/CEIL(C) ppm	mg/m³	OSHA PELs TWA ppm	mg/m³	STEL/CEIL(C) ppm	mg/m³	NIOSH RELs TWA ppm	mg/m³	STEL/CEIL(C) ppm	mg/m³	DFG MAKs TWA ppm	mg/m³	PEAK/CEIL(C) ppm	mg/m³	AIHA WEELs TWA ppm	mg/m³	STEL/CEIL(C) ppm	mg/m³	CARCINOGENICITY CATEGORY
Tetra-n-octyltin compounds, as Sn													0.002*	0.0098 I Skin**; D	II (2)						MAK-4
													*can also be found as vapor **for n-octyltin cmpds whose organic ligands are already designated "Sa" or "Sh", these designations also apply								
Tetrasodium pyro-phosphate 7722-88-5	TLV® withdrawn due to insufficient data									5											
Tetryl 479-45-8		1.5				1.5 Skin				1.5 Skin				Skin; Sh							MAK-3B
Thallium [7440-28-0] **and soluble compounds, as Tl**		0.02 I Skin				0.1 Skin				0.1 Skin											EPA-II
Theobromine 83-67-0																					IARC-3
Theophylline 58-55-9																					IARC-3
Thiabendazole 148-79-8														20 I C; 5	II (2)						
Thimerosal (Sodium ethylmercurithiosalicylate) 54-64-8	See Mercury, aryl compounds									See Mercury, aryl compounds				Sh							

SUBSTANCE / CAS#	ACGIH® TLVs® TWA ppm	ACGIH® TLVs® TWA mg/m³	ACGIH® TLVs® STEL/CEIL(C) ppm	ACGIH® TLVs® STEL/CEIL(C) mg/m³	OSHA PELs TWA ppm	OSHA PELs TWA mg/m³	OSHA PELs STEL/CEIL(C) ppm	OSHA PELs STEL/CEIL(C) mg/m³	NIOSH RELs TWA ppm	NIOSH RELs TWA mg/m³	NIOSH RELs STEL/CEIL(C) ppm	NIOSH RELs STEL/CEIL(C) mg/m³	DFG MAKs TWA ppm	DFG MAKs TWA mg/m³	DFG MAKs PEAK/CEIL(C) ppm	DFG MAKs PEAK/CEIL(C) mg/m³	AIHA WEELs TWA ppm	AIHA WEELs TWA mg/m³	AIHA WEELs STEL/CEIL(C) ppm	AIHA WEELs STEL/CEIL(C) mg/m³	CARCINOGENICITY CATEGORY
Thioacetamide 62-55-5																					IARC-2B NTP-R
4,4'-Thiobis(6-tert-butyl-m-cresol) 96-69-5	1 I				15*; 5** *Total dust **Respirable fraction				10*; 5** *Total dust **Respirable fraction												TLV-A4
4,4'-Thiodianiline 139-65-1																					IARC-2B MAK-2 NTP-R
Thioglycolates													2 I		II (2) Skin; Sh; C						
Thioglycolic acid 68-11-1	1	3.8 Skin							1	4 Skin			Skin; Sh								
Thionyl chloride 7719-09-7			C 0.2								C 1	C 5									
Thiotepa 52-24-4																					IARC-1 NTP-K
Thiouracil 141-90-2																					IARC-2B
Thiourea 62-56-6															Sh; SP						IARC-3 MAK-3B NTP-R

SUBSTANCE CAS#	ACGIH TLVs TWA ppm	ACGIH TLVs TWA mg/m³	ACGIH TLVs STEL/CEIL(C) ppm	ACGIH TLVs STEL/CEIL(C) mg/m³	OSHA PELs TWA ppm	OSHA PELs TWA mg/m³	OSHA PELs STEL/CEIL(C) ppm	OSHA PELs STEL/CEIL(C) mg/m³	NIOSH RELs TWA ppm	NIOSH RELs TWA mg/m³	NIOSH RELs STEL/CEIL(C) ppm	NIOSH RELs STEL/CEIL(C) mg/m³	DFG MAKs TWA ppm	DFG MAKs TWA mg/m³	DFG MAKs PEAK/CEIL(C) ppm	DFG MAKs PEAK/CEIL(C) mg/m³	AIHA WEELs TWA ppm	AIHA WEELs TWA mg/m³	AIHA WEELs STEL/CEIL(C) ppm	AIHA WEELs STEL/CEIL(C) mg/m³	CARCINOGENICITY CATEGORY
Thiram (Tetra-methylthiuram disulfide) 137-26-8		0.05 **IFV** (SEN) NIC-DSEN				5				5				1 **I** Sh; C		II (2)					IARC-3 TLV-A4
Tin, metal 7440-31-5		2				2				2											
Tin, organic compounds, as Sn 7440-31-5		0.1 Skin		0.2		0.1				0.1* *except Cyhexatin Skin				0.1 **I** Skin; D		II (2)					TLV-A4
Tin, oxide and inorganic compounds, except SnH₄, as Sn		2				2* *inorganic compounds except oxides				2											
Tin oxides, as Sn 18282-10-5; 21651-19-4		2								2											
Titanium dioxide 13463-67-7		(10) NIC-1 **R** NIC-A3				15* *Total dust				*See* Pocket Guide App. A											IARC-2B MAK-3A NIOSH-Ca (TLV-A4)
Titanium tetrachloride 7550-45-0																		0.5			
Tobacco, smokeless																					IARC-1 NTP-K
Tolidine, o-isomer (3,3'-Dimethylbenzidine) 119-93-7		Skin								Skin *See* Pocket Guide Apps. A and C		C 0.02* *60-min									IARC-2B TLV-A3 MAK-2 NIOSH-Ca NTP-R

OCCUPATIONAL EXPOSURE VALUES

SUBSTANCE / CAS#	ACGIH® TLVs® TWA ppm	mg/m³	STEL/CEIL(C) ppm	mg/m³	OSHA PELs TWA ppm	mg/m³	STEL/CEIL(C) ppm	mg/m³	NIOSH RELs TWA ppm	mg/m³	STEL/CEIL(C) ppm	mg/m³	DFG MAKs TWA ppm	mg/m³	PEAK/CEIL(C) ppm	mg/m³	AIHA WEELs TWA ppm	mg/m³	STEL/CEIL(C) ppm	mg/m³	CARCINOGENICITY CATEGORY
o-Tolidine-based dyes									minimize exposure; handle with caution See Pocket Guide App. C												NIOSH-Ca
Toluene (Toluol) 108-88-3	20	75 BEI			200		C 300; 500* *10-min peak per 8-hr shift		100	375	150	560	50	190 Skin; C	II (4)						EPA-II IARC-3 TLV-A4
Toluene-2,4- [584-84-9] or 2,6-diisocyanate [91-08-7] (or as a mixture)	(0.005) NIC-0.001* *IFV (SEN) NIC-Skin; DSEN; RSEN; A3	(0.036) 0.007*	(0.02) 0.003*	(0.14) 0.021*			C 0.02 CAS: 584-84-9 only	C 0.14		CAS: 584-84-9 only See Pocket Guide App. A				Sa							IARC-2B* MAK-3A NIOSH-Ca *CAS: 26471-62-5 NTP-R* (TLV-A4)
Toluenesulfonyl chloride, p-isomer 98-59-9																			C 5		
Toluidine hydrochloride, o-isomer 636-21-5																					NTP-R
Toluidine, m-isomer 108-44-1	2	8.8 Skin; BEIₘ																			TLV-A4
Toluidine, o-isomer 95-53-4	2	8.8 Skin; BEIₘ			5	22 Skin			Skin See Pocket Guide App. A				Skin; 3A								IARC-1 MAK-1 NIOSH-Ca NTP-R TLV-A3
Toluidine, p-isomer 106-49-0	2	8.8 Skin; BEIₘ							See Pocket Guide App. A				Skin; Sh								MAK-3B NIOSH-Ca TLV-A3
Toremifene 89778-26-7																					IARC-3

| SUBSTANCE | ACGIH® TLVs® | | | | OSHA PELs | | | | NIOSH RELs | | | | DFG MAKs | | | | AIHA WEELs | | | | CARCINOGENICITY |
| | TWA | | STEL/CEIL(C) | | TWA | | STEL/CEIL(C) | | TWA | | STEL/CEIL(C) | | TWA | | PEAK/CEIL(C) | | TWA | | STEL/CEIL(C) | | |
CAS#	ppm	mg/m³	ppm	mg/m³	ppm	mg/m³	ppm	mg/m³	ppm	mg/m³	ppm	mg/m³	ppm	mg/m³	ppm	mg/m³	ppm	mg/m³	ppm	mg/m³	CATEGORY
Treosulfan 299-75-2																					IARC-1
Tribromochloromethane 594-15-0																					EPA-D
Tribromodiphenyl ether 49690-94-0																					EPA-D
Tributyl phosphate 126-73-8	5 **IFV** BEI_A				5				0.2	2.5			1	11 Skin; C	II (2)						MAK-4 TLV-A3
Tri-n-butyltin compounds, as Sn													0.004*	0.02 **I** Skin**; B *can also be found as vapor **for n-butyltin cmpds whose organic ligands are already designated "Sa" or "Sh", these designations also apply	I (1)						MAK-4
Tributyltin oxide 56-35-9														*See Tri-n-butyltin compounds*							EPA-D; CBD
Trichlormethine (Trimustine hydrochloride) 817-09-4																					IARC-2B
Trichloroacetic acid 76-03-9	(1) NIC-0.5	(6.7) NIC-3.34							1	7											EPA-S IARC-2B TLV-A3

SUBSTANCE / CAS#	ACGIH® TLVs® TWA ppm	ACGIH® TLVs® TWA mg/m³	ACGIH® TLVs® STEL/CEIL(C) ppm	ACGIH® TLVs® STEL/CEIL(C) mg/m³	OSHA PELs TWA ppm	OSHA PELs TWA mg/m³	OSHA PELs STEL/CEIL(C) ppm	OSHA PELs STEL/CEIL(C) mg/m³	NIOSH RELs TWA ppm	NIOSH RELs TWA mg/m³	NIOSH RELs STEL/CEIL(C) ppm	NIOSH RELs STEL/CEIL(C) mg/m³	DFG MAKs TWA ppm	DFG MAKs TWA mg/m³	DFG MAKs PEAK/CEIL(C) ppm	DFG MAKs PEAK/CEIL(C) mg/m³	AIHA WEELs TWA ppm	AIHA WEELs TWA mg/m³	AIHA WEELs STEL/CEIL(C) ppm	AIHA WEELs STEL/CEIL(C) mg/m³	CARCINOGENICITY CATEGORY
Trichloroacetonitrile 545-06-2																					IARC-3
1,2,3-Trichlorobenzene 87-61-6													5	38	II (2) Skin; C						
1,2,4-Trichlorobenzene 120-82-1			C 5	C 37							C 5	C 40			Skin						EPA-D MAK-3B
1,3,5-Trichlorobenzene 108-70-3													5	38	II (2) Skin; C						
2,3,4-Trichloro-1-butene 2431-50-7															Skin						MAK-2
Trichlorocyclopenta-diene 77323-84-3																					EPA-D
1,1,2-Trichloroethane 79-00-5	10	55		Skin	10	45		Skin	10	45	Skin See Pocket Guide Apps. A and C		10	55	II (2) Skin						EPA-C TLV-A3 IARC-3 MAK-3B NIOSH-Ca
Trichloroethylene 79-01-6	10	54	25	135 BEI	100		C 200; 300*	*5-min peak in any 2 hrs	See Pocket Guide Apps. A and C						Skin; 3B						EPA-CaH NTP-R IARC-1 TLV-A2 MAK-1 NIOSH-Ca
Trichlorofluoromethane (Fluorotrichloromethane; FC-11) 75-69-4			C 1000	C 5620	1000	5600					C 1000	C 5600	1000	5700	II (2) C						TLV-A4

SUBSTANCE CAS#	ACGIH® TLVs® TWA ppm	TWA mg/m³	STEL/CEIL(C) ppm	STEL/CEIL(C) mg/m³	OSHA PELs TWA ppm	TWA mg/m³	STEL/CEIL(C) ppm	STEL/CEIL(C) mg/m³	NIOSH RELs TWA ppm	TWA mg/m³	STEL/CEIL(C) ppm	STEL/CEIL(C) mg/m³	DFG MAKs TWA ppm	TWA mg/m³	PEAK/CEIL(C) ppm	PEAK/CEIL(C) mg/m³	AIHA WEELs TWA ppm	TWA mg/m³	STEL/CEIL(C) ppm	STEL/CEIL(C) mg/m³	CARCINOGENICITY CATEGORY
Trichloronaphthalene 1321-65-9		5 Skin				5 Skin				5 Skin				Skin							
2,4,6-Trichlorophenol (Trichlorophenol) 88-06-2																					EPA-B2 NTP-R
2(2,4,5-Trichlorophenoxy)propionic acid (2,4,5-TP) 93-72-1																					EPA-D
1,2,3-Trichloropropane 96-18-4	(10) NIC-0.05 NIC-A2	(60) NIC-0.3		(Skin)	50	300			10 *See* Pocket Guide App. A	60				Skin							EPA-L IARC-2A MAK-2 NIOSH-Ca NTP-R (TLV-A3)
Trichlorosilane 10025-78-2																			C 0.5		
1,1,2-Trichloro-1,2,2-trifluoroethane (CFC-113) 76-13-1	1000	7670	1250	9590	1000	7600			1000	7600	1250	9500	500	3900 D	II (2)						TLV-A4
Trichlorphon 52-68-6		1 **I** BEI₄																			IARC-3 TLV-A4
Triethanolamine 102-71-6		5											5 **I**	D	I (4)						IARC-3
Triethoxysilane 998-30-1																		0.05			

SUBSTANCE / CAS#	ACGIH® TLVs® TWA ppm	ACGIH® TLVs® TWA mg/m³	ACGIH® TLVs® STEL/CEIL(C) ppm	ACGIH® TLVs® STEL/CEIL(C) mg/m³	OSHA PELs TWA ppm	OSHA PELs TWA mg/m³	OSHA PELs STEL/CEIL(C) ppm	OSHA PELs STEL/CEIL(C) mg/m³	NIOSH RELs TWA ppm	NIOSH RELs TWA mg/m³	NIOSH RELs STEL/CEIL(C) ppm	NIOSH RELs STEL/CEIL(C) mg/m³	DFG MAKs TWA ppm	DFG MAKs TWA mg/m³	DFG MAKs PEAK/CEIL(C) ppm	DFG MAKs PEAK/CEIL(C) mg/m³	AIHA WEELs TWA ppm	AIHA WEELs TWA mg/m³	AIHA WEELs STEL/CEIL(C) ppm	AIHA WEELs STEL/CEIL(C) mg/m³	CARCINOGENICITY CATEGORY
Triethylamine 121-44-8	1	4.1	(3) NIC-2 Skin	(12.4) NIC-8.2	25	100							1	4.2 D	I (2)						TLV-A4
Triethylene glycol 112-27-6														1000 I (because formation of a mist is possible, exposure should be minimized) B	II (2)						
Triethylene glycol diacrylate 1680-21-3														Sh				1		Skin	
Triethylene glycol diglycidyl ether 1954-28-5																					IARC-3
Triethylene glycol dimethacrylate 109-16-0														Sh							
Triethylene glycol monomethyl ether 112-35-6														50 I C	II (2)						
Triethylene tetramine 112-24-3														Sh				1	6	Skin	
1,3,5-Triethylhexa-hydro-1,3,5-triazine 7779-27-3																					MAK-3B
Triethyl phosphate 78-40-0																			7.45		

SUBSTANCE CAS#	ACGIH® TLVs® TWA ppm	mg/m³	STEL/CEIL(C) ppm	mg/m³	OSHA PELs TWA ppm	mg/m³	STEL/CEIL(C) ppm	mg/m³	NIOSH RELs TWA ppm	mg/m³	STEL/CEIL(C) ppm	mg/m³	DFG MAKs TWA ppm	mg/m³	PEAK/CEIL(C) ppm	mg/m³	AIHA WEELs TWA ppm	mg/m³	STEL/CEIL(C) ppm	mg/m³	CARCINOGENICITY CATEGORY
Trifluorobromomethane (Bromotrifluoromethane) 75-63-8	1000	6090			1000	6100			1000	6100			1000	6200	II (8) C						
1,1,1-Trifluoroethane 420-46-2																	1000				
2,2,2-Trifluoroethanol 75-89-8																	0.3				
Trifluralin 1582-09-8																					EPA-C IARC-3
1,3,5-Triglycidyl-s-triazinetrione 2451-62-9		0.05																			
Triisobutyl phosphate 126-71-6														Sh							
Trimellitic anhydride 552-30-7	0.0005 **IFV** Skin; (SEN) NIC-DSEN; RSEN		0.002 **IFV**						0.005 handle as extremely toxic substance	0.04				0.04 Sa	I (1)						
Trimethoxysilane 2487-90-3																	0.05				
Trimethylamine 75-50-3	5	12	15	36					10	24	15	36	2	4.9 C	I (2)		1				

SUBSTANCE CAS#	ACGIH® TLVs® TWA ppm	mg/m³	STEL/CEIL(C) ppm	mg/m³	OSHA PELs TWA ppm	mg/m³	STEL/CEIL(C) ppm	mg/m³	NIOSH RELs TWA ppm	mg/m³	STEL/CEIL(C) ppm	mg/m³	DFG MAKs TWA ppm	mg/m³	PEAK/CEIL(C) ppm	mg/m³	AIHA WEELs TWA ppm	mg/m³	STEL/CEIL(C) ppm	mg/m³	CARCINOGENICITY CATEGORY
4,4′,6-Trimethylangelicin plus ultraviolet A radiation 90370-29-9																					IARC-3
2,4,5-Trimethylaniline 137-17-7														Skin							IARC-3 MAK-2
2,4,6-Trimethylaniline 88-05-1																					IARC-3
Trimethyl benzene, all isomers 95-63-6; 108-67-8; 526-73-8	25*	123*							25	125			20	100	II (2) C						
*mixed isomers CAS: 25551-13-7																					
Trimethylchlorosilane 75-77-4																			C 5		
Trimethylolpropane triacrylate 15625-89-5														Sh		Skin		1			
Trimethylolpropane trimethacrylate 3290-92-4																Skin		1			
Trimethylpentane, all isomers 29222-48-8																					MAK-3A
Trimethyl phosphate 512-56-1														Skin; 2							MAK-3B

SUBSTANCE / CAS#	ACGIH® TLVs® TWA ppm	mg/m³	STEL/CEIL(C) ppm	mg/m³	OSHA PELs TWA ppm	mg/m³	STEL/CEIL(C) ppm	mg/m³	NIOSH RELs TWA ppm	mg/m³	STEL/CEIL(C) ppm	mg/m³	DFG MAKs TWA ppm	mg/m³	PEAK/CEIL(C) ppm	mg/m³	AIHA WEELs TWA ppm	mg/m³	STEL/CEIL(C) ppm	mg/m³	CARCINOGENICITY CATEGORY
Trimethyl phosphite 121-45-9	2	10							2	10				Skin							
4,5′,8-Trimethylpsoralen 3902-71-4																					IARC-3
2,4,7-Trinitrofluorenone 129-79-3																					MAK-3B
2,4,6-Trinitrotoluene (TNT) 118-96-7		0.1				1.5				0.5											EPA-C IARC-3 MAK-2
		Skin; BEI$_M$				Skin				Skin				Skin; Sh; 3B							
Tri-n-octyltin compounds, as Sn													0.002*	0.0098 I	II (2)						MAK-4
														Skin**; B							
													*can also be found as vapor **for n-octyltin cmpds whose organic ligands are already designated "Sa" or "Sh", these designations also apply							
Triorthocresyl phosphate 78-30-8		0.1				0.1				0.1											TLV-A4
		Skin; BEI$_A$								Skin											
Triphenyl amine 603-34-9									5												
		TLV® withdrawn due to insufficient data																			
Triphenylene 217-59-4																					IARC-3

SUBSTANCE CAS#	ACGIH® TLVs®				OSHA PELs				NIOSH RELs				DFG MAKs				AIHA WEELs				CARCINOGENICITY CATEGORY
	TWA		STEL/CEIL(C)		TWA		STEL/CEIL(C)		TWA		STEL/CEIL(C)		TWA		PEAK/CEIL(C)		TWA		STEL/CEIL(C)		
	ppm	mg/m³	ppm	mg/m³	ppm	mg/m³	ppm	mg/m³	ppm	mg/m³	ppm	mg/m³	ppm	mg/m³	ppm	mg/m³	ppm	mg/m³	ppm	mg/m³	
Triphenyl phosphate 115-86-6		3				3				3											TLV-A4
Triphenyl phosphine 603-35-0														5 I		II (2) Sh; C					
Tripropylene glycol diacrylate 42978-66-5																Sh					
Trisodium phosphate 7601-54-9																				5	
Trypan Blue 72-57-1																					IARC-2B
Tungsten [7440-33-7] and insoluble compounds, as W		5		10						5		10									
Tungsten, soluble compounds, as W		1		3						1		3									
Tungsten carbide, cemented 11107-01-0; 12718-69-3; 37329-49-0									containing 5–15% Cobalt See Pocket Guide App. C												
Turpentine [8006-64-2] and selected monoterpenes 80-56-8; 127-91-3; 13466-78-9	20	112 (SEN) NIC-DSEN			100	560 CAS: 8006-64-2 only			100	560 CAS: 8006-64-2 only				CAS: 8006-64-2 only Sh							MAK-3A* TLV-A4 *CAS: 8006-64-2 only

SUBSTANCE CAS#	ACGIH® TLVs®				OSHA PELs				NIOSH RELs				DFG MAKs				AIHA WEELs				CARCINOGENICITY CATEGORY
	TWA		STEL/CEIL(C)		TWA		STEL/CEIL(C)		TWA		STEL/CEIL(C)		TWA		PEAK/CEIL(C)		TWA		STEL/CEIL(C)		
	ppm	mg/m³	ppm	mg/m³	ppm	mg/m³	ppm	mg/m³	ppm	mg/m³	ppm	mg/m³	ppm	mg/m³	ppm	mg/m³	ppm	mg/m³	ppm	mg/m³	
1-Undecanethiol (Undecyl mercaptan) 5332-52-5											C 0.5*	C 3.9* *15-min									
Uracil mustard 66-75-1																					IARC-2B
Uranium, natural [7440-61-1], **soluble and in-soluble compounds, as U**	0.2			0.6	0.05* 0.25**				0.05* 0.2**			0.6**	The threshold value of the Commission on Radiological Protection of 20 mSv per year or 400 mSv per working lifetime corresponds to about 25 µg uranium/m3 for poorly soluble uranium cmpds and 250 µg uranium/m3 for soluble cmpds (MMAD of 5 µm). Skin; 3A								MAK-2 NIOSH-Ca TLV-A1
		BEI			*Soluble; **Insoluble				*Soluble; **Insoluble See Pocket Guide App. A												
Urea 57-13-6																	10				EPA-II
Urethane (Carbamic acid, ethyl ester; Ethyl carbamate) 51-79-6													Skin; 3A								IARC-2A MAK-2 NTP-R
n-Valeraldehyde 110-62-3	50	176							50	175			See Pocket Guide App. C								
Vanadium [7440-62-2] **and inorganic compounds**													Inhalable fraction 2								MAK-2
Vanadium pentoxide, as V 1314-62-1	0.05 I						C 0.5* C 0.1**				C 0.05*					2					IARC-2B MAK-2 TLV-A3
					*Respirable dust, as V₂O₅ **Fume, as V₂O₅				*15-min, except Vanadium metal and Vanadium carbide												

SUBSTANCE / CAS#	ACGIH® TLVs® TWA ppm	mg/m³	STEL/CEIL(C) ppm	mg/m³	OSHA PELs TWA ppm	mg/m³	STEL/CEIL(C) ppm	mg/m³	NIOSH RELs TWA ppm	mg/m³	STEL/CEIL(C) ppm	mg/m³	DFG MAKs TWA ppm	mg/m³	PEAK/CEIL(C) ppm	mg/m³	AIHA WEELs TWA ppm	mg/m³	STEL/CEIL(C) ppm	mg/m³	CARCINOGENICITY CATEGORY
Vanillin 121-33-5																		10			
Vat Yellow 4 128-66-5																					IARC-3
Vegetable oil mist	TLV® withdrawn due to insufficient data				15*; 5**				10*; 5**												
					*Total dust **Respirable fraction				*Total dust **Respirable fraction												
Vinblastine sulfate 143-67-9																					IARC-3
Vincristine sulfate 2068-78-2																					IARC-3
Vinyl acetate 108-05-4	10	35	15	53							C 4*										IARC-2B MAK-3A TLV-A3
											*15-min										
Vinyl bromide 593-60-2	0.5	2.2							See Pocket Guide App. A												IARC-2A NIOSH-Ca NTP-R TLV-A2
Vinylcarbazole 1484-13-5													Sh								
Vinyl chloride (Chloroethylene) 75-01-4	1	2.6			1		5*														EPA-K; A NTP-K IARC-1 OSHA-Ca MAK-1 TLV-A1 NIOSH-Ca
					*avg. not exceeding any 15 min See 29 CFR 1910.1017				See Pocket Guide App. A												

SUBSTANCE / CAS#	ACGIH® TLVs® TWA ppm	mg/m³	STEL/CEIL(C) ppm	mg/m³	OSHA PELs TWA ppm	mg/m³	STEL/CEIL(C) ppm	mg/m³	NIOSH RELs TWA ppm	mg/m³	STEL/CEIL(C) ppm	mg/m³	DFG MAKs TWA ppm	mg/m³	PEAK/CEIL(C) ppm	mg/m³	AIHA WEELs TWA ppm	mg/m³	STEL/CEIL(C) ppm	mg/m³	CARCINOGENICITY CATEGORY
Vinyl chloride-Vinyl acetate copolymers 9003-22-9																					IARC-3
4-Vinyl cyclohexene 100-40-3	0.1	0.44													Skin		1	4.4			IARC-2B MAK-2 TLV-A3
Vinyl cyclohexene dioxide 106-87-6	0.1	0.57 Skin							10	60 Skin *See* Pocket Guide App. A					Skin						IARC-2B TLV-A3 MAK-2 NIOSH-Ca NTP-R
Vinyl fluoride 75-02-5	1	1.9							1		C 5 *See* 29 CFR 1910.1017										IARC-2A NTP-R TLV-A2
Vinylidene chloride (1,1-Dichloroethylene) 75-35-4	5	20								*See* Pocket Guide App. A			2	8	II (2) C						EPA-I*; MAK-3B S**; C NIOSH-Ca IARC-3 TLV-A4 *oral route; **inhalation
Vinylidene chloride-Vinyl chloride copolymers 9011-06-7																					IARC-3
Vinylidene fluoride (1,1-Difluoroethylene) 75-38-7	500	1310							1		C 5 Use 29 CFR 1910.1017										IARC-3 MAK-3B TLV-A4
N-Vinyl-2-pyrrolidone 88-12-0	0.05	0.23													Skin						IARC-3 MAK-2 TLV-A3
Vinyl toluene 25013-15-4	50	242	100	483	100	480			100	480			100	490	I (2)						IARC-3 TLV-A4

SUBSTANCE / CAS#	ACGIH® TLVs® TWA ppm	mg/m³	STEL/CEIL(C) ppm	mg/m³	OSHA PELs TWA ppm	mg/m³	STEL/CEIL(C) ppm	mg/m³	NIOSH RELs TWA ppm	mg/m³	STEL/CEIL(C) ppm	mg/m³	DFG MAKs TWA ppm	mg/m³	PEAK/CEIL(C) ppm	mg/m³	AIHA WEELs TWA ppm	mg/m³	STEL/CEIL(C) ppm	mg/m³	CARCINOGENICITY CATEGORY
Vinyltrichlorosilane 75-94-5																			C 1		
Vitamin K substances 12001-79-5																					IARC-3
VM & P naphtha 8032-32-4	TLV® withdrawn; refer to Appendix H								350		C 1800*										TLV-A3
									*15-min												
Warfarin 81-81-2	0.1				0.1				0.1				0.0016*	0.02 **I**	II (8)						
												*can also be found as vapor; Skin; B								
Welding fumes, not otherwise specified									for Welding fumes See Pocket Guide App. A												IARC-2B NIOSH-Ca
Wollastonite 13983-17-0																					IARC-3
Wood dusts, beech and oak	1 **I**								See Wood dusts, all other species												IARC-1 MAK-1 NTP-K TLV-A1
Wood dusts, birch, mahogany, teak, walnut	1 **I**								See Wood dusts, all other species												IARC-1 MAK-3B NTP-K TLV-A2
Wood dusts, all other species	1 **I**								1 for Wood dust See Pocket Guide App. A												IARC-1 NIOSH-Ca NTP-K TLV-A4

SUBSTANCE / CAS#	ACGIH® TLVs® TWA ppm	mg/m³	STEL/CEIL(C) ppm	mg/m³	OSHA PELs TWA ppm	mg/m³	STEL/CEIL(C) ppm	mg/m³	NIOSH RELs TWA ppm	mg/m³	STEL/CEIL(C) ppm	mg/m³	DFG MAKs TWA ppm	mg/m³	PEAK/CEIL(C) ppm	mg/m³	AIHA WEELs TWA ppm	mg/m³	STEL/CEIL(C) ppm	mg/m³	CARCINOGENICITY CATEGORY
Wood dusts, softwood	1 I								*See* Wood dusts, all other species												IARC-1 MAK-3B NTP-K TLV-A4
Wood dusts, western red cedar	0.5 I												includes African white wood								IARC-1 MAK-3B NTP-K TLV-A4
	(SEN) NIC-DSEN; RSEN								*See* Wood dusts, all other species				Sah								
Xylanases 37278-89-0													Sa								
Xylene (Dimethylbenzene), o-, m-, p-isomers 95-47-6; 106-42-3; 108-38-3; 1330-20-7	100	434	150	651	100	435			100	435	150	655	100	440	II (2)						EPA-I IARC-3 TLV-A4
	BEI												Skin; D								
m-Xylene α,α′-diamine 1477-55-0			C 0.1								C 0.1										
	Skin								Skin				Sh								
Xylidine, mixed isomers 87-59-2; 95-64-7; 108-69-0; 1300-73-8	0.5 IFV		2.5 IFV		5	25			2	10			isomers except the 2,4- and 2,6-isomers								MAK-3A TLV-A3
	Skin; BEI_M				Skin				Skin				Skin								
2,4-Xylidine 95-68-1													Skin								IARC-3 MAK-2
2,5-Xylidine 95-78-3													Skin								IARC-3 MAK-3A
2,6-Xylidine (2,6-Dimethylaniline) 87-62-7													Skin								IARC-2B MAK-2

SUBSTANCE / CAS#	ACGIH® TLVs® TWA ppm	TWA mg/m³	STEL/CEIL(C) ppm	mg/m³	OSHA PELs TWA ppm	TWA mg/m³	STEL/CEIL(C) ppm	mg/m³	NIOSH RELs TWA ppm	TWA mg/m³	STEL/CEIL(C) ppm	mg/m³	DFG MAKs TWA ppm	TWA mg/m³	PEAK/CEIL(C) ppm	mg/m³	AIHA WEELs TWA ppm	TWA mg/m³	STEL/CEIL(C) ppm	mg/m³	CARCINOGENICITY CATEGORY
Yellow AB 85-84-7																					IARC-3
Yellow OB 131-79-3																					IARC-3
Yttrium [7440-65-5] **and compounds, as Y**	1				1				1												
Zalcitabine 7481-89-2																					IARC-2B
Zectran 315-18-4																					IARC-3
Zeolites, excluding erionite 1318-02-1																					IARC-3
Zidovudine (AZT) 30516-87-1																					IARC-2B
Zinc and compounds 7440-66-6															0.1 **R** 2 **I**	I (4)* I (2)** inorganic compounds *Respirable **Inhalable, excluding Zinc chloride					EPA-II; D; I

SUBSTANCE / CAS#	ACGIH® TLVs® TWA ppm	TWA mg/m³	STEL/CEIL(C) ppm	STEL/CEIL(C) mg/m³	OSHA PELs TWA ppm	TWA mg/m³	STEL/CEIL(C) ppm	STEL/CEIL(C) mg/m³	NIOSH RELs TWA ppm	TWA mg/m³	STEL/CEIL(C) ppm	STEL/CEIL(C) mg/m³	DFG MAKs TWA ppm	TWA mg/m³	PEAK/CEIL(C) ppm	PEAK/CEIL(C) mg/m³	AIHA WEELs TWA ppm	TWA mg/m³	STEL/CEIL(C) ppm	STEL/CEIL(C) mg/m³	CARCINOGENICITY CATEGORY
Zinc beryllium silicate, as Be 39413-47-3	*See* Beryllium and compounds, as Be				0.002		C 0.005 0.025* *30-min peak per 8-hr shift				C 0.0005 *See* Pocket Guide App. A		Sah								EPA-B1; CBD**; K* IARC-1 MAK-1 NIOSH-Ca NTP-K TLV-A1 *inhaled; **ingested
Zinc chloride, fume 7646-85-7	1			2	1				1			2		0.1 R 2 I *Respirable	I (1)* I (4)** **Inhalable						EPA-II
Zinc chromates, as Cr 11103-86-9; 13530-65-9; 37300-23-5	0.01					0.005*	C 0.1** *CAS: 13530-65-9 only **as CrO₃, CAS: 11103-86-9 and 37300-23-5				*See* Chromic acid and chromates		*See* Chromium (VI) inorganic compounds, insoluble								IARC-1 NTP-K TLV-A1
Zinc oxide 1314-13-2		2 R		10 R		15*; 5** *Total dust **Respirable fraction				5 Dust only		C 15		0.1 R 2 I *Respirable	I (4)* I (2)** **Inhalable						EPA-II; D; I
Zinc oxide, fume 1314-13-2						5				5		10		0.1 R 2 I *Respirable	I (4)* I (2)** **Inhalable						EPA-II; D; I
Zinc pyrithione 13463-41-7														Skin							
Zinc stearate 557-05-1	10					15*; 5** *Total dust **Respirable fraction			10*; 5**		*Total dust **Respirable fraction			0.1 R 2 I *Respirable	I (4)* I (2)** **Inhalable						EPA-II; D; I TLV-A4
Zineb 12122-67-7																					IARC-3
Ziram 137-30-4																					IARC-3

SUBSTANCE / CAS#	ACGIH® TLVs® TWA ppm	ACGIH® TLVs® TWA mg/m³	ACGIH® TLVs® STEL/CEIL(C) ppm	ACGIH® TLVs® STEL/CEIL(C) mg/m³	OSHA PELs TWA ppm	OSHA PELs TWA mg/m³	OSHA PELs STEL/CEIL(C) ppm	OSHA PELs STEL/CEIL(C) mg/m³	NIOSH RELs TWA ppm	NIOSH RELs TWA mg/m³	NIOSH RELs STEL/CEIL(C) ppm	NIOSH RELs STEL/CEIL(C) mg/m³	DFG MAKs TWA ppm	DFG MAKs TWA mg/m³	DFG MAKs PEAK/CEIL(C) ppm	DFG MAKs PEAK/CEIL(C) mg/m³	AIHA WEELs TWA ppm	AIHA WEELs TWA mg/m³	AIHA WEELs STEL/CEIL(C) ppm	AIHA WEELs STEL/CEIL(C) mg/m³	CARCINOGENICITY CATEGORY
Zirconium, elemental 7440-67-7		5		10										1 I Sah; D		I (1)					TLV-A4
Zirconium [7440-67-7] compounds, as Zr		5		10		5				5 except Zirconium tetrachloride		10									TLV-A4
Zirconium [7440-67-7], insoluble compounds										5 except Zirconium tetrachloride		10		1 I Sah; D		I (1)					
Zirconium [7440-67-7], soluble compounds										5 except Zirconium tetrachloride		10		Sah							

50-00-0	Formaldehyde
50-07-7	Mitomycin C
50-18-0	Cyclophosphamide
50-29-3	DDT (Dichlorodiphenyltrichloroethane)
50-32-8	Benzo[a]pyrene
50-33-9	Phenylbutazone
50-41-9	Clomiphene citrate
50-44-2	6-Mercaptopurine
50-53-3	Chlorpromazine
50-55-5	Reserpine
50-76-0	Actinomycin D
50-78-2	Acetylsalicylic acid (Aspirin)
51-02-5	Pronetalol hydrochloride
51-03-6	Piperonyl butoxide
51-18-3	2,4,6-tris(1-Aziridinyl)-s-triazine
51-21-8	5-Fluorouracil
51-52-5	Propylthiouracil
51-75-2	Nitrogen mustard (N-Methyl-bis[2-chloroethyl] amine)
51-79-6	Urethane (Carbamic acid, ethyl ester; Ethyl carbamate)
52-01-7	Spironolactone
52-24-4	Thiotepa
52-46-0	Apholate
52-51-7	2-Bromo-2-nitro-1,3-propanediol
52-68-6	Trichlorphon
53-03-2	Prednisone
53-70-3	Dibenz[a,h]anthracene
53-96-3	2-Acetylaminofluorene (2-AAF)
54-05-7	Chloroquine
54-11-5	Nicotine
54-31-9	Furosemide (Frusemide)
54-64-8	Thimerosal (Sodium ethylmercurithiosalicylate)
54-85-3	Isonicotinic acid hydrazine (Isoniazid)
55-18-5	N-Nitrosodiethylamine (NDEA)

55-38-9	Fenthion
55-63-0	Nitroglycerin (NG)
55-86-7	Nitrogen mustard hydrochloride (Mechlorethamine hydrochloride)
55-98-1	1,4-Butanediol dimethanesulfonate (Busulphan; Myleran®)
56-04-2	Methylthiouracil
56-23-5	Carbon tetrachloride (Tetrachloromethane)
56-25-7	Cantharidin
56-35-9	Tributyltin oxide
56-38-2	Parathion
56-53-1	Diethylstilboestrol
56-55-3	Benz[a]anthracene
56-72-4	Coumaphos
56-75-7	Chloramphenicol
56-81-5	Glycerin
57-06-7	Allyl isothiocyanate
57-12-5	Cyanide, free
57-13-6	Urea
57-14-7	1,1-Dimethylhydrazine
57-24-9	Strychnine
57-39-6	tris(2-Methyl-1-aziridinyl)phosphine oxide
57-41-0	Phenytoin
57-50-1	Sucrose
57-55-6	Propylene glycol
57-57-8	β-Propiolactone
57-68-1	Sulfamethazine
57-74-9	Chlordane
57-88-5	Cholesterol
58-08-2	Caffeine
58-14-0	Pyrimethamine
58-55-9	Theophylline
58-89-9	Lindane (γ-Hexachlorocyclohexane)
58-93-5	Hydrochlorothiazide
59-05-2	Methotrexate

74-93-1	Methyl mercaptan (Methanethiol)
74-96-4	Ethyl bromide (Bromoethane)
74-97-5	Chlorobromomethane (Bromochloromethane)
74-98-6	Propane
74-99-7	Methyl acetylene (Propyne)
75-00-3	Ethyl chloride (Chloroethane)
75-01-4	Vinyl chloride (Chloroethylene)
75-02-5	Vinyl fluoride
75-04-7	Ethylamine
75-05-8	Acetonitrile
75-07-0	Acetaldehyde (Acetic aldehyde)
75-08-1	Ethyl mercaptan (Ethanethiol)
75-09-2	Dichloromethane (Methylene chloride)
75-10-5	Difluoromethane
75-12-7	Formamide
75-15-0	Carbon disulfide
75-18-3	Dimethyl sulfide
75-21-8	Ethylene oxide (EtO)
75-25-2	Bromoform (Tribromomethane)
75-27-4	Bromodichloromethane
75-28-5	Isobutane [see Butane, all isomers]
75-29-6	2-Chloropropane
75-31-0	Isopropylamine
75-34-3	1,1-Dichloroethane (Ethylidene chloride)
75-35-4	Vinylidene chloride (1,1-Dichloroethylene)
75-36-5	Acetyl chloride
75-37-6	1,1-Difluoroethane
75-38-7	Vinylidene fluoride (1,1-Difluoroethylene)
75-43-4	Dichlorofluoromethane (FC-21)
75-44-5	Phosgene (Carbonyl chloride)
75-45-6	Chlorodifluoromethane (FC-22)
75-47-8	Iodoform
75-50-3	Trimethylamine

75-52-5	Nitromethane
75-55-8	Propyleneimine (2-Methylaziridine)
75-56-9	Propylene oxide (1,2-Epoxypropane)
75-60-5	Cacodylic acid
75-61-6	Difluorodibromomethane
75-62-7	Bromotrichloromethane
75-63-8	Trifluorobromomethane (Bromotrifluoromethane)
75-65-0	tert-Butanol (tert-Butyl alcohol)
75-68-3	1-Chloro-1,1-difluoroethane (FC-142b)
75-69-4	Trichlorofluoromethane (Fluorotrichloromethane; FC-11)
75-71-8	Dichlorodifluoromethane (FC-12)
75-72-9	Chlorotrifluoromethane (FC-13)
75-74-1	Tetramethyl lead, as Pb
75-77-4	Trimethylchlorosilane
75-78-5	Dimethyldichlorosilane
75-79-6	Methyltrichlorosilane
75-83-2	2,2-Dimethyl butane [see Hexane, isomers, other than n-Hexane]
75-84-3	Neopentyl alcohol [see Pentanol, all isomers]
75-85-4	2-Methyl-2-butanol [see Pentanol, all isomers]
75-86-5	Acetone cyanohydrin
75-87-6	Chloral
75-88-7	2-Chloro-1,1,1-trifluoroethane
75-89-8	2,2,2-Trifluoroethanol
75-94-5	Vinyltrichlorosilane
75-99-0	2,2-Dichloropropionic acid
76-01-7	Pentachloroethane
76-03-9	Trichloroacetic acid
76-06-2	Chloropicrin (Trichloronitromethane)
76-11-9	1,1,1,2-Tetrachloro-2,2-difluoroethane (FC-112a)
76-12-0	1,1,2,2-Tetrachloro-1,2-difluoroethane (FC-112)
76-13-1	1,1,2-Trichloro-1,2,2-trifluoroethane (CFC-113)
76-14-2	Dichlorotetrafluoroethane (1,2-Dichloro-1,1,2,2-tetrafluoroethane)
76-15-3	Chloropentafluoroethane

CAS Number	Chemical Name
83-79-4	Rotenone, commercial
84-15-1	Terphenyl, o-isomer [see Terphenyl, o-, m-, p-isomers]
84-65-1	Anthraquinone
84-66-2	Diethyl phthalate
84-74-2	Dibutyl phthalate
85-00-7	Diquat dibromide [see Diquat]
85-01-8	Phenanthrene
85-42-7	Hexahydrophthalic anhydride, all isomers
85-44-9	Phthalic anhydride
85-68-7	Butyl benzyl phthalate
85-83-6	Scarlet Red
85-84-7	Yellow AB
85-86-9	Sudan III
86-30-6	N-Nitrosodiphenylamine
86-50-0	Azinphos-methyl
86-54-4	Hydralazine
86-57-7	1-Nitronaphthalene
86-73-7	Fluorene
86-74-8	Carbazole
86-88-4	ANTU (α-Naphthylthiourea)
87-29-6	Cinnamyl anthranilate
87-59-2	2,3-Xylidine [see Xylidine, mixed isomers]
87-61-6	1,2,3-Trichlorobenzene
87-62-7	2,6-Xylidine (2,6-Dimethylaniline)
87-68-3	Hexachlorobutadiene
87-86-5	Pentachlorophenol
88-05-1	2,4,6-Trimethylaniline
88-06-2	2,4,6-Trichlorophenol (Trichlorophenol)
88-10-8	Diethylcarbamoyl chloride
88-12-0	N-Vinyl-2-pyrrolidone
88-72-2	Nitrotoluene, o-isomer (2-Nitrotoluene)
88-73-3	Nitrochlorobenzene, o-isomer (2-Chloronitrobenzene)
88-85-7	Dinoseb
88-88-0	Picryl chloride
88-89-1	Picric acid (2,4,6-Trinitrophenol)
89-72-5	o-sec-Butylphenol
90-04-0	Anisidine, o-isomer
90-12-0	1-Methyl naphthalene
90-30-2	N-Phenyl-1-naphthylamine
90-43-7	Phenylphenol, o-isomer
90-65-3	Penicillic acid
90-94-8	Michler's ketone
91-08-7	Toluene-2,6-diisocyanate
91-15-6	Phthalodinitrile, o-isomer
91-20-3	Naphthalene
91-22-5	Quinoline
91-23-6	2-Nitroanisole
91-29-2	4-Nitro-4'-aminodiphenylamine-2-sulfonic acid
91-57-6	2-Methylnaphthalene [see 1-Methylnaphthalene and 2-Methylnaphthalene]
91-59-8	β-Naphthylamine (2-Naphthylamine)
91-64-5	Coumarin
91-93-0	3,3'-Dimethoxybenzidine-4,4'-diisocyanate
91-94-1	3,3'-Dichlorobenzidine
91-95-2	3,3'-Diaminobenzidine
92-06-8	Terphenyl, m-isomer [see Terphenyl, o-, m-, p-isomers]
92-52-4	Biphenyl (Diphenyl)
92-67-1	4-Aminodiphenyl
92-84-2	Phenothiazine
92-87-5	Benzidine
92-93-3	4-Nitrodiphenyl (4-Nitrobiphenyl)
92-94-4	Terphenyl, p-isomer [see Terphenyl, o-, m-, p-isomers]
93-15-2	Methyleugenol
93-72-1	2(2,4,5-Trichlorophenoxy)propionic acid (2,4,5-TP)
93-76-5	2,4,5-T (2,4,5-Trichlorophenoxyacetic acid)
94-36-0	Benzoyl peroxide (Dibenzoyl peroxide)

94-37-1	Dipentamethylene-thiuram disulfide
94-58-6	Dihydrosafrole
94-59-7	Safrole
94-75-7	2,4-D (2,4-Dichlorophenoxyacetic acid)
95-06-7	Sulfallate
95-13-6	Indene
95-33-0	N-Cyclohexyl-2-benzothiazolesulfenamide
95-47-6	Xylene, o-isomer (1,2-Dimethylbenzene) [see Xylene (Dimethylbenzene), o-, m-, p-isomers]
95-48-7	Cresol, o-isomer [see Cresol, all isomers]
95-49-8	Chlorotoluene, o-isomer
95-50-1	Dichlorobenzene, o-isomer (1,2-Dichlorobenzene)
95-51-2	Chloroaniline, o-isomer
95-53-4	Toluidine, o-isomer
95-54-5	Phenylenediamine, o-isomer
95-63-6	1,2,4-Trimethylbenzene [see Trimethyl benzene, all isomers]
95-64-7	3,4-Xylidine [see Xylidine, mixed isomers]
95-68-1	2,4-Xylidine
95-69-2	4-Chloro-o-toluidine
95-70-5	2,5-Diaminotoluene (Toluene-2,5-diamine)
95-76-1	3,4-Dichloroaniline
95-78-3	2,5-Xylidine
95-79-4	5-Chloro-o-toluidine
95-80-7	2,4-Diaminotoluene (Toluene-2,4-diamine)
95-83-0	4-Chloro-o-phenylenediamine
96-09-3	Styrene-7,8-oxide (1,2-Epoxyethylbenzene)
96-12-8	1,2-Dibromo-3-chloropropane (DBCP)
96-13-9	2,3-Dibromo-1-propanol
96-14-0	3-Methylpentane [see Hexane, isomers, other than n-Hexane]
96-18-4	1,2,3-Trichloropropane
96-22-0	Diethyl ketone
96-23-1	1,3-Dichloro-2-propanol
96-24-2	3-Monochloro-1,2-propanediol
96-29-7	Methyl ethyl ketoxime (2-Butanone oxime)
96-33-3	Methyl acrylate (Acrylic acid, methyl ester)
96-34-4	Chloroacetic acid, methyl ester (Methyl chloroacetate)
96-37-7	Methylcyclopentane [see Hexane, isomers, other than n-Hexane]
96-45-7	Ethylene thiourea
96-48-0	γ-Butyrolactone
96-69-5	4,4'-Thiobis(6-tert-butyl-m-cresol)
97-00-7	1-Chloro-2,4-dinitrobenzene
97-18-7	Bithionol
97-53-0	Eugenol
97-54-1	Isoeugenol and its isomers
97-56-3	o-Aminoazotoluene
97-63-2	Ethyl methacrylate (Methylacrylic acid, ethyl ester)
97-77-8	Disulfiram
97-88-1	n-Butyl methacrylate
97-90-5	Ethylene glycol dimethacrylate
97-99-4	Tetrahydrofurfuryl alcohol
98-00-0	Furfuryl alcohol
98-01-1	Furfural
98-07-7	Benzotrichloride (Benzyl trichloride)
98-29-3	p-tert-Butylcatechol (4-[1,1-Dimethylethyl]-1,2-benzenediol)
98-51-1	p-tert-Butyltoluene
98-54-4	p-tert-Butylphenol
98-57-7	p-Chlorophenyl methyl sulfone
98-59-9	Toluenesulfonyl chloride, p-isomer
98-73-7	4-tert-Butylbenzoic acid
98-82-8	Cumene
98-83-9	α-Methyl styrene
98-86-2	Acetophenone
98-87-3	Benzal chloride (Benzyl dichloride)
98-88-4	Benzoyl chloride
98-95-3	Nitrobenzene
99-08-1	Nitrotoluene, m-isomer (3-Nitrotoluene)

CAS Number	Chemical Name
99-54-7	3,4-Dichloronitrobenzene
99-55-8	5-Nitro-o-toluidine (4-Nitro-2-aminotoluene)
99-56-9	1,2-Diamino-4-nitrobenzene
99-57-0	2-Amino-4-nitrophenol
99-59-2	5-Nitro-o-anisidine
99-65-0	Dinitrobenzene, m-isomer [see Dinitrobenzene, all isomers]
99-80-9	N-Methyl-N,4-dinitrosoaniline
99-96-7	Hydroxybenzoic acid
99-97-8	N,N-Dimethyl-p-toluidine
99-99-0	Nitrotoluene, p-isomer (4-Nitrotoluene)
100-00-5	Nitrochlorobenzene, p-isomer (4-Chloronitrobenzene)
100-01-6	Nitroaniline, p-isomer
100-21-0	Terephthalic acid (p-Phthalic acid)
100-25-4	Dinitrobenzene, p-isomer [see Dinitrobenzene, all isomers]
100-37-8	2-Diethylaminoethanol
100-40-3	4-Vinyl cyclohexene
100-41-4	Ethyl benzene
100-42-5	Styrene, monomer (Phenylethylene; Vinyl benzene)
100-44-7	Benzyl chloride
100-51-6	Benzyl alcohol
100-52-7	Benzaldehyde
100-61-8	N-Methyl aniline (Monomethyl aniline)
100-63-0	Phenylhydrazine
100-74-3	N-Ethylmorpholine
100-75-4	N-Nitrosopiperidine (NPIP)
100-97-0	Hexamethylenetetramine
101-14-4	4,4'-Methylene bis(2-chloroaniline) (MBOCA)
101-21-3	Chloropropham
101-25-7	Dinitrosopentamethylenetetramine
101-54-2	4-Aminodiphenylamine
101-55-3	p-Bromodiphenyl ether
101-61-1	4,4'-Methylene bis(N,N'-dimethyl)aniline (Michler's base)
101-68-8	Methylene bisphenyl isocyanate (MDI; Diphenylmethane-4,4'-diisocyanate)
101-72-4	N-Isopropyl-N'-phenyl-p-phenylenediamine
101-77-9	4,4'-Methylene dianiline (4,4'-Diaminodiphenyl-methane)
101-80-4	bis(4-Aminophenyl)ether (4,4'-Oxydianiline; 4,4'-Diaminodiphenyl ether)
101-83-7	Dicyclohexylamine
101-84-8	Phenyl ether, vapor
101-87-1	N-Cyclohexyl-N'-phenyl-p-phenylenediamine
101-90-6	Diglycidyl resorcinol ether
102-50-1	Cresidine, m-isomer
102-54-5	Dicyclopentadienyl iron, as Fe (Ferrocene)
102-71-6	Triethanolamine
102-77-2	2-(4-Morpholinylmercapto)benzothiazole
102-81-8	2-N-Dibutylaminoethanol
103-03-7	Phenicarbazide
103-11-7	2-Ethylhexyl acrylate (Acrylic acid, 2-ethylhexyl ester)
103-23-1	Di(2-ethylhexyl)adipate
103-33-3	Azobenzene
103-71-9	Phenyl isocyanate
103-90-2	Acetaminophen (Paracetamol)
104-12-1	4-Chlorophenyl isocyanate
104-54-1	Cinnamyl alcohol
104-55-2	Cinnamaldehyde
104-76-7	2-Ethylhexanol
104-94-9	Anisidine, p-isomer
105-11-3	Benzoquinone dioxime, p-isomer
105-46-4	sec-Butyl acetate
105-55-5	N,N'-Diethylthiourea
105-60-2	Caprolactam
105-74-8	Lauroyl peroxide
106-24-1	Geraniol
106-35-4	Ethyl butyl ketone (3-Heptanone)
106-42-3	Xylene, p-isomer (1,4-Dimethylbenzene) [see Xylene (Dimethyl

108-65-6	1-Methoxypropyl-2-acetate (Propylene glycol monomethyl ether acetate)
108-67-8	1,3,5-Trimethylbenzene [see Trimethyl benzene, all isomers]
108-69-0	3,5-Xylidine [see Xylidine, mixed isomers]
108-70-3	1,3,5-Trichlorobenzene
108-78-1	Melamine
108-80-5	Isocyanuric acid
108-83-8	Diisobutyl ketone (2,6-Dimethyl-4-heptanone)
108-84-9	sec-Hexyl acetate
108-86-1	Bromobenzene
108-87-2	Methylcyclohexane
108-88-3	Toluene (Toluol)
108-89-4	4-Picoline
108-90-7	Chlorobenzene (Monochlorobenzene)
108-91-8	Cyclohexylamine
108-93-0	Cyclohexanol
108-94-1	Cyclohexanone
108-95-2	Phenol
108-98-5	Phenyl mercaptan
108-99-6	3-Picoline
109-06-8	2-Picoline
109-16-0	Triethylene glycol dimethacrylate
109-17-1	Tetraethylene glycol dimethacrylate
109-53-5	iso-Butyl vinyl ether
109-59-1	2-Isopropoxyethanol (Ethylene glycol isopropyl ether)
109-60-4	n-Propyl acetate
109-66-0	Pentane, all isomers
109-69-3	1-Chlorobutane
109-73-9	n-Butylamine
109-74-0	n-Butyronitrile
109-77-3	Malononitrile
109-79-5	n-Butyl mercaptan (Butanethiol)
109-86-4	2-Methoxyethanol (EGME)

109-87-5	Methylal (Dimethoxymethane)
109-89-7	Diethylamine
109-94-4	Ethyl formate (Formic acid, ethyl ester)
109-99-9	Tetrahydrofuran
110-00-9	Furan
110-01-0	Tetrahydrothiophene (THT)
110-12-3	Methyl isoamyl ketone (Methyl-2-hexanone)
110-19-0	Isobutyl acetate
110-43-0	Methyl n-amyl ketone (2-Heptanone)
110-49-6	2-Methoxyethyl acetate (EGMEA)
110-54-3	n-Hexane (Hexane)
110-57-6	1,4-Dichlorobutene, trans-isomer
110-61-2	Succinonitrile
110-62-3	n-Valeraldehyde
110-65-6	Butynediol
110-66-7	Pentyl mercaptan
110-80-5	2-Ethoxyethanol (EGEE; Cellosolve)
110-82-7	Cyclohexane
110-83-8	Cyclohexene
110-85-0	Piperazine
110-86-1	Pyridine
110-89-4	Piperidine
110-91-8	Morpholine
111-15-9	2-Ethoxyethyl acetate (EGEEA; Cellosolve acetate)
111-27-3	n-Hexyl alcohol
111-30-8	Glutaraldehyde
111-31-9	n-Hexyl mercaptan (n-Hexanethiol)
111-40-0	Diethylene triamine
111-42-2	Diethanolamine
111-44-4	Dichloroethyl ether (bis[2-Chloroethyl]ether)
111-46-6	Diethylene glycol
111-65-9	n-Octane [see Octane, all isomers]
111-66-0	1-Octene

121-88-0	2-Amino-5-nitrophenol
121-91-5	Phthalic acid, m-isomer (Isophthalate)
122-34-9	Simazine
122-39-4	Diphenylamine
122-40-7	α-Amylcinnamaldehyde
122-42-9	Propham
122-60-1	Phenyl glycidyl ether (PGE)
122-66-7	Hydrazobenzene (1,2-Diphenylhydrazine)
122-99-6	2-Phenoxyethanol (Ethylene glycol monophenyl ether)
123-09-1	p-Chlorophenyl methyl sulfide
123-19-3	Dipropyl ketone
123-30-8	p-Aminophenol
123-31-9	Hydroquinone (Dihydroxybenzene)
123-33-1	Maleic hydrazide
123-38-6	Propionaldehyde
123-42-2	Diacetone alcohol (4-Hydroxy-4-methyl-2-pentanone)
123-51-3	Isoamyl alcohol
123-54-6	2,4-Pentanedione
123-72-8	Butyraldehyde
123-73-9	trans-Crotonaldehyde [see Crotonaldehyde]
123-75-1	Pyrrolidine
123-86-4	n-Butyl acetate
123-91-1	1,4-Dioxane (Diethylene dioxide)
123-92-2	Isopentyl acetate (Isoamyl acetate)
124-02-7	Diallylamine
124-04-9	Adipic acid
124-09-4	1,6-Hexanediamine
124-17-4	Butyl carbitol acetate (Diethylene glycol monobutyl ether acetate)
124-38-9	Carbon dioxide
124-40-3	Dimethylamine
124-48-1	Chlorodibromomethane
124-58-3	Methylarsonic acid
124-64-1	Tetrakis(hydroxymethyl)phosphonium chloride

126-07-8	Griseofulvin
126-71-6	Triisobutyl phosphate
126-73-8	Tributyl phosphate
126-72-7	tris(2,3-Dibromopropyl) phosphate
126-85-2	Nitrogen mustard N-oxide
126-98-7	Methylacrylonitrile
126-99-8	β-Chloroprene (2-Chloro-1,3-butadiene)
127-00-4	1-Chloro-2-propanol
127-07-1	Hydroxyurea
127-18-4	Tetrachloroethylene (Perchloroethylene)
127-19-5	N,N-Dimethylacetamide
127-69-5	Sulfafurazole (Sulfisoxazole)
127-91-3	β-Pinene [see Turpentine and selected monoterpenes]
128-37-0	Butylated hydroxytoluene (BHT; 2,6-Di-tert-butyl-p-cresol)
128-66-5	Vat Yellow 4
129-00-0	Pyrene
129-06-6	Sodium warfarin [see Warfarin]
129-15-7	2-Methyl-1-nitroanthraquinone, uncertain purity
129-16-8	Merbromin
129-17-9	Blue VRS
129-20-4	Oxyphenbutazone
129-43-1	1-Hydroxyanthraquinone
129-79-3	2,4,7-Trinitrofluorenone
131-11-3	Dimethylphthalate
131-79-3	Yellow OB
132-27-4	Sodium-o-phenylphenate
132-32-1	3-Amino-9-ethylcarbazole
132-64-9	Dibenzofuran
133-06-2	Captan
133-07-3	Folpet
134-29-2	Anisidine hydrochloride, o-isomer
134-32-7	α-Naphthylamine (1-Naphthylamine)
135-20-6	Cupferron

135-88-6	N-Phenyl-β-naphthylamine
136-35-6	Diazaminobenzene
136-40-3	Phenazopyridine hydrochloride
136-78-7	Sesone (Sodium-2,4-dichlorophenoxyethyl sulfate)
137-05-3	Methyl 2-cyanoacrylate
137-17-7	2,4,5-Trimethylaniline
137-26-8	Thiram (Tetramethylthiuram disulfide)
137-30-4	Ziram
137-32-6	2-Methyl-1-butanol [see Pentanol, all isomers]
138-22-7	n-Butyl lactate
138-59-0	Shikimic acid
138-86-3	DL-Limonene
139-05-9	Sodium cyclamate
139-13-9	Nitrilotriacetic acid
139-65-1	4,4′-Thiodianiline
139-94-6	Nithiazide
140-11-4	Benzyl acetate
140-56-7	p-Dimethylaminoazobenzenediazo sodium sulfonate
140-57-8	Aramite®
140-88-5	Ethyl acrylate (Acrylic acid, ethyl ester)
141-32-2	n-Butyl acrylate (Acrylic acid ester, n-Butyl ester)
141-37-7	3,4-Epoxy-6-methylcyclohexylmethyl-3,4-epoxy-6-methyl-cyclohexane carboxylate
141-43-5	Ethanolamine (2-Aminoethanol)
141-66-2	Dicrotophos
141-78-6	Ethyl acetate
141-79-7	Mesityl oxide
141-90-2	Thiouracil
142-64-3	Piperazine dihydrochloride
142-82-5	n-Heptane [see Heptane, all isomers]
142-83-6	2,4-Hexadienal
143-07-7	Lauric acid
143-10-2	Decylmercaptan
143-33-9	Sodium cyanide, as CN
143-50-0	Chlordecone
143-67-9	Vinblastine sulfate
144-34-3	Methyl selenac
144-62-7	Oxalic acid
148-01-6	3,5-Dinitro-o-toluamide (Dinitolmide)
148-18-5	Sodium diethyldithiocarbamate
148-24-3	8-Hydroxyquinoline
148-79-8	Thiabendazole
148-82-3	Melphalan
149-29-1	Patulin
149-30-4	2-Mercaptobenzothiazole
149-57-5	2-Ethylhexanoic acid
150-13-0	p-Aminobenzoic acid
150-68-5	Monuron
150-69-6	Dulcin
150-76-5	4-Methoxyphenol
151-50-8	Potassium cyanide, as CN
151-56-4	Ethyleneimine
151-67-7	Halothane
154-93-8	bis(Chloroethyl)nitrosourea (BCNU)
156-10-5	p-Nitrosodiphenylamine
156-51-4	Phenelzine sulfate
156-59-2	cis-1,2-Dichloroethylene [see 1,2-Dichloroethylene, all isomers]
156-60-5	trans-1,2-Dichloroethylene [see 1,2-Dichloroethylene, all isomers]
156-62-7	Calcium cyanamide
189-55-9	Dibenzo[a,i]pyrene
189-64-0	Dibenzo[a,h]pyrene
191-07-1	Coronene
191-24-2	Benzo[ghi]perylene
191-26-4	Anthanthrene
191-30-0	Dibenzo[a,l]pyrene

192-47-2	Dibenzo[h,rst]pentaphene
192-51-8	Dibenzo[e,l]pyrene
192-65-4	Dibenzo[a,e]pyrene
192-97-2	Benzo[e]pyrene
193-09-9	Naphtho[2,3-e]pyrene
193-39-5	Indeno[1,2,3,cd]pyrene
194-59-2	7H-Dibenzo[c,g]carbazole
195-19-7	Benzo[c]phenanthrene
196-78-1	Benzo[g]chrysene
198-55-0	Perylene
202-94-8	11H-Benz[bc]aceanthrylene
202-98-2	4H-Cyclopenta[def]chrysene
203-12-3	Benzo[ghi]fluoranthene
203-20-3	Naphtho[2,1-a]fluoranthene
203-33-5	Benz[j]aceanthrylene
203-33-8	Benzo[a]fluoranthene
205-12-9	Benzo[c]fluorene
205-82-3	Benzo[j]fluoranthene
205-99-2	Benzo[b]fluoranthene
206-44-0	Fluoranthene
207-08-9	Benzo[k]fluoranthene
207-83-0	13H-Dibenzo[a,g]fluorene
208-96-8	Acenaphthylene
211-91-6	Benz[l]aceanthrylene
213-46-7	Picene
214-17-5	Benzo[b]chrysene
215-58-7	Dibenz[a,c]anthracene
217-59-4	Triphenylene
218-01-9	Chrysene
224-41-9	Dibenz[a,j]anthracene
224-42-0	Dibenz[a,j]acridine
224-53-3	Dibenz[c,h]acridine
225-11-6	Benz[a]acridine

225-51-4	Benz[c]acridine
226-36-8	Dibenz[a,h]acridine
238-84-6	Benzo[a]fluorene
239-35-0	Benzo[b]naphtho[2,1-d]-thiophene
243-17-4	Benzo[b]fluorene
262-12-4	Dibenzo-p-dioxin
271-89-6	Benzofuran
287-92-3	Cyclopentane
298-00-0	Methyl parathion
298-02-2	Phorate
298-04-4	Disulfoton
298-81-7	8-Methoxypsoralen(Methoxsalen) plus ultraviolet A radiation
299-75-2	Treosulfan
299-84-3	Ronnel
299-86-5	Crufomate
300-76-5	Naled (Dibrom; Dimethyl-1,2-dibromo-2,2-dichloroethyl-phosphate)
302-01-2	Hydrazine
302-17-0	Chloral hydrate
303-34-4	Lasiocarpine
303-47-9	Ochratoxin A
305-03-3	Chlorambucil
306-83-2	2,2-Dichloro-1,1,1-trifluoroethane (FC-123)
309-00-2	Aldrin
311-45-5	Diethyl-p-nitrophenyl phosphate
313-67-7	Aristolochic acid
314-13-6	Evans Blue
314-40-9	Bromacil
315-18-4	Zectran
315-22-0	Monocrotaline
319-84-6	α-Hexachlorocyclohexan
319-85-7	β-Hexachlorocyclohexane [see 1,2,3,4,5,6-Hexachlorocyclohexane, mixture of isomers]

CAS Number	Name
541-41-3	Ethyl chloroformate (Chloroformic acid ethyl ester)
541-73-1	Dichlorobenzene, m-isomer
541-85-5	Ethyl amyl ketone (5-Methyl-3-heptanone)
542-56-3	Isobutyl nitrite
542-75-6	1,3-Dichloropropene
542-78-9	Malonaldehyde
542-88-1	bis(Chloromethyl)ether
542-92-7	Cyclopentadiene
543-27-1	Isobutyl chloroformate [see Chloroformic acid butyl ester]
545-06-2	Trichloroacetonitrile
545-55-1	tris(1-Aziridinyl)-phosphine oxide
546-93-0	Magnesite
551-74-6	Mannomustine dihydrochloride
552-30-7	Trimellitic anhydride
555-84-0	1-[(5-Nitrofurfurylidene)amino]-2-imidazolidinone
556-52-5	Glycidol (2,3-Epoxy-1-propanol)
556-88-7	Nitroguanidine
557-05-1	Zinc stearate
558-13-4	Carbon tetrabromide
562-10-7	Doxylamine succinate
563-12-2	Ethion
563-41-7	Semicarbazide hydrochloride
563-47-3	3-Chloro-2-methylpropene
563-80-4	Methyl isopropyl ketone (MIPK)
565-59-3	2,3-Dimethylpentane [see Heptane, all isomers]
569-61-9	CI Basic Red 9
581-89-5	2-Nitronaphthalene
583-60-8	o-Methylcyclohexanone
584-02-1	3-Pentanol [see Pentanol, all isomers]
584-84-9	Toluene-2,4-diisocyanate (TDI)
589-34-4	3-Methylhexane [see Heptane, all isomers]
590-18-1	cis-2-Butene [see Butenes, all isomers]
590-35-2	2,2-Dimethylpentane [see Heptane, all isomers]
591-27-5	3-Aminophenol
591-76-4	2-Methylhexane [see Heptane, all isomers]
591-78-6	Methyl n-butyl ketone (2-Hexanone)
592-01-8	Calcium cyanide, as CN
592-34-7	Chloroformic acid butyl ester (n-Butyl chloroformate)
592-41-6	1-Hexene
592-45-0	1,4-Hexadiene
592-62-1	Methylazoxymethanol acetate
593-60-2	Vinyl bromide
593-70-4	Chlorofluoromethane (FC-31)
594-15-0	Tribromochloromethane
594-18-3	Dibromodichloromethane
594-42-3	Perchloromethyl mercaptan
594-72-9	1,1-Dichloro-1-nitroethane
598-55-0	Methyl carbamate
598-56-1	N,N-Dimethylethylamine
598-75-4	D-3-Methyl-2-butanol [see Pentanol, all isomers]
598-78-7	2-Chloropropionic acid
600-25-9	1-Chloro-1-nitropropane
601-77-4	N-Nitrosodiisopropylamine
602-60-8	9-Nitroanthracene
602-87-9	5-Nitroacenaphthene
603-34-9	Triphenyl amine
603-35-0	Triphenyl phosphine
604-75-1	Oxazepam
606-20-2	2,6-Dinitrotoluene
607-57-8	2-Nitrofluorene
608-73-1	Hexachlorocyclohexane, technical (t-HCH)
608-93-5	Pentachlorobenzene
609-20-1	2,6-Dichloro-p-phenylenediamine
612-00-0	Dowtherm® Q
612-64-6	N-Nitrosoethylphenylamine
612-83-9	3,3′-Dichlorobenzidine dihydrochloride

872-50-4	N-Methyl-2-pyrrolidone
892-21-7	3-Nitrofluoranthene
915-67-3	Amaranth
919-86-8	Demeton-S-methyl
920-37-6	2-Chloroacrylonitrile
923-26-2	2-Hydroxypropyl methacrylate (Methacrylic acid 2-hydroxypropyl ester)
924-16-3	N-Nitrosodi-n-butylamine (DBN)
930-55-2	N-Nitrosopyrrolidine (NPYR)
934-73-6	p-Chlorophenyl methyl sulfoxide
944-22-9	Fonofos
950-37-8	Methidathion
989-38-8	Rhodamine 6G
994-05-8	tert-Amyl methyl ether (TAME)
996-35-0	N,N-Dimethylisopropylamine
998-30-1	Triethoxysilane
999-61-1	2-Hydroxypropyl acrylate
1024-57-3	Heptachlor epoxide
1070-70-8	1,4-Butanediol diacrylate
1072-52-2	2-(1-Aziridinyl)ethanol
1116-54-7	N-Nitrosodiethanolamine (NDELA)
1120-71-4	Propane sultone (1,3-Propane sultone)
1121-03-5	2,4-Butane sultone
1143-38-0	Dithranol
1163-19-5	Decabromodiphenyl oxide
1189-85-1	tert-Butyl chromate, as CrO_3
1239-45-8	Ethidium bromide
1300-73-8	Xylidine, mixed isomers
1302-74-5	Emery
1303-00-0	Gallium arsenide
1303-28-2	Arsenic pentoxide, as As
1303-86-2	Boron oxide
1303-96-4	Sodium tetraborate, decahydrate

1304-82-1	Bismuth telluride, Undoped; Bismuth telluride, Se-doped, as Bi_2Te_3
1305-62-0	Calcium hydroxide
1305-78-8	Calcium oxide
1306-38-3	Cerium oxide and cerium compounds
1307-79-9	Terbufos
1309-37-1	Iron oxide (Fe_2O_3)
1309-48-4	Magnesium oxide
1309-64-4	Antimony trioxide, as Sb
1310-58-3	Potassium hydroxide
1310-65-2	Lithium hydroxide
1310-73-2	Sodium hydroxide
1313-27-5	Molybdenum trioxide
1313-99-1	Nickel oxide
1314-06-3	Nickel sesquioxide
1314-13-2	Zinc oxide; Zinc oxide, fume
1314-56-3	Phosphorus pentoxide
1314-61-0	Tantalum oxide, dusts, as Ta
1314-62-1	Vanadium pentoxide, as V
1314-80-3	Phosphorus pentasulfide
1317-43-7	Nemalite, fibrous dust
1317-60-8	Hematite
1317-65-3	Calcium carbonate (Limestone; Marble)
1317-95-9	Silica, crystalline, tripoli
1318-02-1	Zeolites, excluding erionite
1319-77-3	Cresol, all isomers
1321-64-8	Pentachloronaphthalene
1321-65-9	Trichloronaphthalene
1321-74-0	Divinyl benzene
1327-33-9	Antimony oxide
1327-53-3	Arsenic trioxide, as As
1330-20-7	Xylene (Dimethylbenzene)
1330-43-4	Sodium tetraborate, anhydrous

2179-59-1	Allyl propyl disulfide
2224-44-4	4-(2-Nitrobutyl)-morpholine (70% w/v) [see 4-(2-Nitrobutyl) morpholine (70% w/v)/4,4'-(2-Ethyl-2-nitro-1,3-propanediyl)bis morpholine (20% w/v) mixture]
2234-13-1	Octachloronaphthalene
2238-07-5	Diglycidyl ether (DGE)
2243-62-1	1,5-Naphthalenediamine
2303-16-4	Diallate
2318-18-5	Senkirkine
2353-45-9	Fast Green FCF
2358-84-1	Diethylene glycol dimethacrylate
2381-21-7	1-Methylpyrene
2385-85-5	Mirex
2386-90-5	bis(2,3-Epoxycyclopentyl)ether
2402-79-1	2,3,5,6-Tetrachloropyridine
2425-06-1	Captafol
2425-79-8	1,4-Butanediol diglycidyl ether
2425-85-6	CI Pigment Red 3
2426-08-6	n-Butyl glycidyl ether (BGE)
2429-74-5	CI Direct Blue 15
2431-50-7	2,3,4-Trichloro-1-butene
2432-99-7	11-Aminoundecanoic acid
2443-39-2	9,10-Epoxystearic acid, cis-isomer
2451-62-9	1,3,5-Triglycidyl-s-triazinetrione
2455-24-5	Tetrahydrofurfuryl methacrylate
2465-27-2	Auramine hydrochloride
2475-45-8	Disperse Blue 1
2487-90-3	Trimethoxysilane
2527-58-4	2,2'-Dithiobis(N-methylbenzamide)
2528-36-1	Dibutyl phenyl phosphate
2551-62-4	Sulfur hexafluoride
2634-33-5	1,2-Benzisothiazol-3(2H)-one
2646-17-5	Oil Orange SS
2682-20-4	2-Methyl-2,3-dihydroisothiazol-3-one
2698-41-1	Chlorobenzylidene malononitrile, o-isomer
2699-79-8	Sulfuryl fluoride
2757-90-6	Agaritine
2764-72-9	Diquat
2783-94-0	Sunset Yellow FCF
2784-94-3	HC Blue No. 1
2807-30-9	2-Propoxyethanol (Ethylene glycol mono-n-propyl ether)
2832-19-1	Chloroacetamide-N-methylol (CAM)
2832-40-8	Disperse Yellow 3
2835-39-4	Allyl isovalerate
2837-89-0	2-Chloro-1,1,1,2-tetrafluoroethane
2855-13-2	3-Aminomethyl-3,5,5-trimethyl cyclohexylamine (Isophorone diamine)
2871-01-4	HC Red No. 3
2872-52-8	Disperse Red 1
2885-00-9	Octadecyl mercaptan
2917-26-2	Cetylmercaptan (1-Hexadecanethiol)
2921-88-2	Chlorpyrifos
2955-38-6	Prazepam
2971-90-6	Clopidol
2973-10-6	Diisopropyl sulfate
3018-12-0	Dichloroacetonitrile
3033-62-3	bis(2-Dimethylaminoethyl)ether (DMAEE)
3033-77-0	Glycidyl trimethyl ammonium chloride
3068-88-0	β-Butyrolactone
3101-60-8	p-tert-Butyl phenol glycidyl ether
3118-97-6	Sudan II
3165-93-3	p-Chloro-o-toluidine hydrochloride
3173-72-6	1,5-Naphthylene diisocyanate (NDI)
3179-89-3	Disperse Red 17
3252-43-5	Dibromoacetonitrile
3290-92-4	Trimethylolpropane trimethacrylate

6358-64-1	2,5-Dimethoxy-4-chloroaniline
6368-72-5	Sudan Red 7B
6373-74-6	CI Acid Orange 3
6385-62-2	Diquat dibromide monohydrate [see Diquat]
6416-57-5	Sudan Brown RR
6419-19-8	Aminotris(methylenephosphonic acid)
6423-43-4	Propylene glycol dinitrate (PGDN)
6440-58-0	1,3-Dimethylol-5,5-dimethyl hydantoin
6459-94-5	CI Acid Red 114
6870-67-3	Jacobine
6923-22-4	Monocrotophos
7085-85-0	Ethyl cyanoacrylate (Ethyl 2-cyanoacrylate)
7099-43-6	5,6-Cyclopenteno-1,2-benzanthracene
7411-49-6	3,3′-Diaminobenzidine tetrahydrochloride
7429-90-5	Aluminum, metal and insoluble compounds
7439-92-1	Lead and inorganic compounds, as Pb
7439-96-5	Manganese, and inorganic compounds, as Mn; Manganese, fume, as Mn
7439-97-6	Mercury, aryl compounds, as Hg; Mercury, elemental and inorganic compounds, as Hg
7439-98-7	Molybdenum and insoluble compounds, as Mo; Molybdenum, soluble compounds, as Mo
7440-01-9	Neon
7440-02-0	Nickel compounds; Nickel elemental; Nickel insoluble compounds, as Ni; Nickel soluble compounds, as Ni
7440-06-4	Platinum, metal; Platinum, soluble salts, as Pt
7440-07-5	Plutonium
7440-16-6	Rhodium, elemental
7440-21-3	Silicon
7440-22-4	Silver, metal
7440-25-7	Tantalum, metal
7440-28-0	Thallium and soluble compounds, as Tl
7440-31-5	Tin, metal
7440-33-7	Tungsten and insoluble compounds, as W
7440-36-0	Antimony and compounds, as Sb
7440-37-1	Argon
7440-38-2	Arsenic and inorganic compounds (except arsine), as As
7440-39-3	Barium and soluble compounds, as Ba
7440-41-7	Beryllium and compounds, as Be
7440-42-8	Boron and compounds
7440-43-9	Cadmium and compounds, as Cd; Cadmium and inorganic compounds
7440-47-3	Chromium (III) inorganic compounds, as Cr; Chromium metal
7440-48-4	Cobalt and compounds; Cobalt and inorganic compounds, as Co; Cobalt with tungsten carbide
7440-50-8	Copper dusts and mists, as Cu; Copper fume, as Cu; Copper and its organic compounds
7440-57-5	Gold and inorganic compounds
7440-58-6	Hafnium and compounds, as Hf
7440-59-7	Helium
7440-61-1	Uranium, natural, soluble and insoluble compounds, as U
7440-62-2	Vanadium and inorganic compounds
7440-65-5	Yttrium and compounds, as Y
7440-66-6	Zinc and compounds
7440-67-7	Zirconium, elemental; Zirconium compounds, as Zr; Zirconium insoluble compounds; Zirconium soluble compounds
7440-74-6	Indium and compounds, as In
7446-09-5	Sulfur dioxide
7446-27-7	Lead phosphate
7446-34-6	Selenium sulfide
7460-84-6	Glycidyl stearate
7481-89-2	Zalcitabine
7487-94-7	Mercuric chloride
7496-02-8	6-Nitrochrysene
7519-36-0	N-Nitrosoproline
7550-45-0	Titanium tetrachloride

7790-98-9	Perchlorate and perchlorate salts
7791-03-9	Lithium perchlorate, anhydrous [see Perchlorate and perchlorate salts]
7803-49-8	Hydroxylamine (and its salts)
7803-51-2	Phosphine
7803-52-3	Antimony hydride (Stibine)
7803-57-8	Hydrazine hydrate and hydrazine salts
7803-62-5	Silicon tetrahydride (Silane)
8001-35-2	Chlorinated camphene (Toxaphene)
8001-50-1	Terpene polychlorinates
8001-58-9	Creosotes
8002-05-9	Petroleum distillates, Naphtha (Rubber solvent)
8002-26-4	Tall oil, distilled
8002-74-2	Paraffin wax fume
8003-34-7	Pyrethrum
8004-13-5	Phenyl ether/biphenyl mixture, vapor
8006-61-9	Gasoline
8006-64-2	Turpentine [see Turpentine and selected monoterpenes]
8008-20-6	Kerosene [see Kerosene/Jet fuels as total hydrocarbon vapor]
8012-95-1	Oil mist, mineral
8018-01-7	Mancozeb
8018-07-3	Acriflavinium chloride
8022-00-2	Methyl demeton (Demeton-methyl)
8030-30-6	Naphtha, coal tar
8032-32-4	VM & P naphtha
8047-67-4	Saccharated iron oxide
8050-09-7	Rosin core solder thermal decomposition products (Colophony)
8052-41-3	Stoddard solvent
8052-42-4	Asphalt fume (Bitumen)
8065-48-3	Demeton
9000-07-1	Carrageenan, native
9001-00-7	Bromelain
9001-73-4	Papain

9001-75-6	Pepsin
9002-84-0	Polytetrafluoroethylene
9002-86-2	Polyvinyl chloride (PVC)
9002-88-4	Polyethylene
9002-89-5	Polyvinyl alcohol
9003-01-4	Polyacrylic acid
9003-04-7	Acrylic acid polymer, neutralized, cross-linked
9003-07-0	Polypropylene
9003-20-7	Polyvinyl acetate
9003-22-9	Vinyl chloride–Vinyl acetate copolymers
9003-31-0	Natural rubber latex, as inhalable allergenic proteins
9003-39-8	Polyvinyl pyrrolidone
9003-53-6	Polystyrene
9003-54-7	Styrene-acrylonitrile copolymers
9003-55-8	Styrene-butadiene copolymers
9004-34-6	Cellulose
9004-51-7	Iron-dextrin complex
9004-66-4	Iron-dextran complex
9005-25-8	Starch
9006-04-6	Natural rubber latex, as inhalable allergenic proteins
9009-54-5	Polyurethane foams
9010-98-4	Polychloroprene
9011-06-7	Vinylidene chloride–Vinyl chloride copolymers
9011-14-7	Polymethyl methacrylate
9014-01-1	Subtilisin Carlsberg [see Subtilisins]
9016-87-9	Polymethylene polyphenyl isocyanate (Polymeric MDI)
10024-97-2	Nitrous oxide
10025-67-9	Sulfur monochloride
10025-78-2	Trichlorosilane
10025-87-3	Phosphorus oxychloride
10026-04-7	Tetrachlorosilane
10026-13-8	Phosphorus pentachloride
10028-15-6	Ozone

13494-80-9	Tellurium and compounds, as Te
13530-65-9	Zinc chromates, as Cr
13552-44-8	4,4′-Methylenedianiline dihydrochloride
13756-19-0	Calcium chromate, as Cr
13838-16-9	Enflurane
13909-09-6	1-(2-Chloroethyl)-3-(4-methylcyclohexyl)-1-nitrosourea (Methyl-CCNU; Semustine)
13952-84-6	sec-Butylamine
13983-17-0	Wollastonite
14166-21-3	Hexahydrophthalic anhydride, trans-isomer [see Hexahydrophthalic anhydride, all isomers]
14464-46-1	Silica, crystalline, cristobalite
14484-64-1	Ferbam
14548-60-8	Benzylhemiformal
14596-37-3	Phosphorus-32
14807-96-6	Talc, containing no asbestos fibers
14808-60-7	Silica, crystalline, α-quartz
14857-34-2	Dimethylethoxysilane
14861-17-7	4-(2,4-Dichlorophenoxy)benzenamine
14901-08-7	Cycasin
14977-61-8	Chromyl chloride
15086-94-9	Eosin
15096-52-3	Sodium aluminum fluoride, as F
15141-18-1	Disperse Blue 124 [see Disperse Blue 106/124]
15159-40-7	N-Chloroformylmorpholine
15468-32-3	Silica, crystalline, tridymite
15501-74-3	Sepiolite, fibrous dust
15503-86-3	Isatidine
15541-45-4	Bromate
15625-89-5	Trimethylolpropane triacrylate
15663-27-1	Cisplatin
15721-02-5	2,2′,5,5′-Tetrachlorobenzidine
15922-78-8	Sodium pyrithione
15972-60-8	Alachlor
16065-83-1	Chromium (III)
16096-31-4	Diglycidyl hexanediol
16219-75-3	Ethylidene norbornene
16543-55-8	N′-Nitrosonornicotine (NNN)
16568-02-8	Gyromitrin
16752-77-5	Methomyl
16812-54-7	Nickel sulfide
16842-03-8	Cobalt hydrocarbonyl, as Co
17117-34-9	3-Nitrobenzanthrone
17702-41-9	Decaborane
17804-35-2	Benomyl
17831-71-9	Tetraethylene glycol diacrylate
18282-10-5	Stannic oxide [see Tin oxides, as Sn]
18307-23-8	Sepiolite
18454-12-1	Lead chromate oxide
18540-29-9	Chromium (VI)
18883-66-4	Streptozotocin
19044-88-3	Oryzalin
19287-45-7	Diborane
19408-74-3	1,2,3,7,8,9-Hexachlorodibenzo-p-dioxin [see Hexachlorodibenzo-p-dioxin, mixture (HxCDD)
19430-93-4	Perfluorobutyl ethylene (PFBE)
19624-22-7	Pentaborane
20073-24-9	3-Carbethoxypsoralen
20268-51-3	7-Nitrobenz[a]anthracene
20589-63-3	3-Nitroperylene
20706-25-6	2-Propoxyethyl acetate (Ethylene glycol monopropyl ether acetate)
20816-12-0	Osmium tetroxide
20830-81-3	Daunomycin
20941-65-5	Ethyl telluric
21087-64-9	Metribuzin
21351-79-1	Cesium hydroxide
21645-51-2	Aluminum hydroxide
21651-19-4	Tin oxide, as Sn

30516-87-1	Zidovudine (AZT)
30560-19-1	Acephate
30618-84-9	Glyceryl monothioglycolate
30899-19-5	Pentanol, all isomers
31027-31-3	4-Isopropylphenyl isocyanate
31242-93-0	o-Chlorinated diphenyl oxide [see Chlorinated diphenyl oxide]
31565-23-8	Di(tert-dodecyl)pentasulfide
32534-81-9	Pentabromodiphenyl ether
32536-52-0	Octabromodiphenyl ether
33229-34-4	HC Blue No. 2
33419-42-0	Etoposide
33543-31-6	2-Methylfluoranthene
34590-94-8	(2-Methoxymethylethoxy)propanol (DPGME)
35074-77-2	Hexamethylene bis(3-[3,5-di-tert-butyl-4-hydroxyphenyl] propionate
35400-43-2	Sulprofos
35691-65-7	1,2-Dibromo-2,4-dicyanobutane
37278-89-0	Xylanases
37300-23-5	Zinc Yellow [see Zinc chromates, as Cr]
37329-49-0	Tungsten carbide, mixed with Co and Ti (78% : 14% : 8%)
37620-20-5	N'-Nitrosoanabasine (NAB)
37971-36-1	2-Phosphono-1,2,4-butanetricarboxylic acid
38571-73-2	1,2,3-tris(Chloromethoxy)propane
39148-24-8	Fosetyl-al
39156-41-7	2,4-Diaminoanisole sulfate
39413-47-3	Zinc beryllium silicate, as Be
39638-32-9	bis-(2-Chloroisopropyl)ether
40088-47-9	Tetrabromodiphenyl ether
40762-15-0	Doxefazepam
41683-62-9	1,2-Dichloromethoxyethane
41851-50-7	Chlorocyclopentadiene
42397-64-8	1,6-Dinitropyrene
42397-65-9	1,8-Dinitropyrene
42978-66-5	Tripropylene glycol diacrylate
49690-94-0	Tribromodiphenyl ether
51218-45-2	Metolachlor
51264-14-3	Amsacrine
51481-61-9	Cimetidine
51630-58-1	Fenvalerate
52645-53-1	Permethrin
52918-63-5	Deltamethrin
53469-21-9	Chlorodiphenyl, 42% chlorine
53973-98-1	Carrageenan, degraded
54208-63-8	Bisphenyl F diglycidyl ether (o,o'-isomer)
54749-90-5	Chlorozotocin
54839-24-6	1-Ethoxy-2-propyl acetate
55290-64-7	Dimethipin
55406-53-6	3-Iodo-2-propynyl butylcarbamate
55557-01-2	N-Nitrosoguvacine
55557-02-3	N-Nitrosoguvacoline
55566-30-8	Tetrakis(hydroxymethyl)phosphonium sulfate
55720-99-5	Chlorinated diphenyl oxide
56894-91-8	1,4-bis(Chloromethoxymethyl)benzene
57018-52-7	1-tert-Butoxy-2-propanol
57117-31-4	2,3,4,7,8-Pentachlorodibenzofuran
57465-28-8	3,4,5,3',4'-Pentachlorobiphenyl (PCB-126)
57469-07-5	Bisphenyl F diglycidyl ether (o,p'-isomer)
57653-85-7	1,2,3,6,7,8-Hexachlorodibenzo-p-dioxin [see Hexachlorodibenzo-p-dioxin, mixture]
57835-92-4	4-Nitropyrene [see Nitropyrenes]
59277-89-3	Aciclovir
59536-65-1	Polybrominated biphenyls (PBBs)
59820-43-8	HC Yellow No. 4
59865-13-3	Cyclosporin A
60102-37-6	Pentasitenine

60153-49-3 3-(Methylnitrosamino)propionitrile (3-[N-Nitrosomethylamino]propionitrile)

60348-60-9 2,2′,4,4′,5-Pentabromodiphenyl ether (BDE-99)

60568-05-0 Furmecyclox

60676-86-0 Silica, amorphous, fused

61788-32-7 Hydrogenated terphenyls

61789-36-4 Calcium naphthenate [see Naphthenate, Na-, Ca-, K-]

61790-13-4 Sodium naphthenate [see Naphthenate, Na-, Ca-, K-]

61790-53-2 Silica, amorphous, diatomaceous earth, uncalcined

61951-51-7 Disperse Blue 124 [see Disperse Blue 106/124]

62450-06-0 3-Amino-1,4-dimethyl-5H-pyrido[4,3-b]indole (Trp-P-1)

62450-07-1 3-Amino-1-methyl-5H-pyrido[4,3-b]indole (Trp-P-2)

62765-93-9 NIAX® Catalyst ESN

63021-86-3 Nitropyrene [see Nitropyrenes]

63041-90-7 6-Nitrobenzo[a]pyrene

63936-56-1 Nonabromodiphenyl ether

64091-90-3 4-(N-Nitrosomethylamino)-4-(3-pyridyl)-1-butanal (NNA)

64091-91-4 4-(N-Nitrosomethylamino)-1-(3-pyridyl)-1-butanone

64742-47-8 Petroleum distillates, hydrotreated light

64742-48-9 Naphtha, petroleum, hydrotreated, heavy

64742-81-0 Hydrosulfurized kerosene [see Kerosene/Jet fuels as total hydrocarbon vapor]

65271-80-9 Mitoxantrone

65996-93-2 Coal tar pitch volatiles, as benzene soluble aerosol

65997-15-1 Portland cement

66072-08-0 Potassium naphthenate [see Naphthenate, Na-, Ca-, K-]

66204-44-2 N,N′-Methylene-bis(5-methyloxazolidine)

66603-10-9 Cyclohexylhydroxydiazene-1-oxide, potassium salt

66733-21-9 Erionite, fibrous dust

67730-10-3 2-Aminodipyrido[1,2-a:3′,2′-d]imidazole (Glu-P-2)

67730-11-4 2-Amino-6-methyldipyrido[1,2-a:3′,2′-d]imidazole (Glu-P-1)

67747-09-5 Prochloraz

68006-83-7 2-Amino-3-methyl-9H-pyrido[2,3-b]indole(MeA-α-C)

68308-34-9 Shale-oils

68334-30-5 Diesel oil [see Diesel fuel]

68359-37-5 Cyfluthrin

68425-15-0 Polysulfides, di-tert-dodecyl [see Di(tert-dodecyl)polysulfides]

68476-30-2 Fuel oil No. 2 [see Diesel fuel]

68476-34-6 Diesel fuel No. 2 [see Diesel fuel]

68476-85-7 L.P.G. (Liquefied petroleum gas)

68516-81-4 Disperse Blue 106/124

68583-56-2 tert-Dodecyl mercaptan, sulfur reaction product [see Di(tert-dodecyl)polysulfides]

68895-54-9 Silica, amorphous, diatomaceous earth, calcined

68916-96-1 Mate, absolute (Tea oil)

68987-42-8 Dowtherm® Q

69012-64-2 Silica, amorphous, silica fume

69655-05-6 Didanosine

70657-70-4 2-Methoxypropyl-1-acetate (Propylene glycol 2-methyl ether-1-acetate)

71267-22-6 N′-Nitrosoanatabine (NAT)

72178-02-0 Fomesafen

73459-03-7 5-Methylangelicin plus ultraviolet A radiation

74115-24-5 Apollo

74222-97-2 Sulfometuron methyl

75321-19-6 1,3,6-Trinitropyrene [see Nitropyrenes]

75321-20-9 1,3-Dinitropyrene

76180-96-6 2-Amino-3-methylimidazo[4,5-f]quinoline (IQ)

76578-14-8 Assure

77094-11-2 2-Amino-3,4-dimethylimidazo[4,5-f]quinoline (MeIQ)

77323-84-3 Trichlorocyclopentadiene

77439-76-0 3-Chloro-4-(dichloromethyl)-5-hydroxy-2(5H)-furanone

77500-04-0 2-Amino-3,8-dimethylimidazo[4,5-f]quinoxaline (MeIQx)

77536-66-4 Actinolite [see Asbestos, all forms]

77536-67-5 Anthophyllite [see Asbestos, all forms]

77536-68-6 Tremolite [see Asbestos, all forms]

77650-28-3	Diesel fuel, marine [see Diesel fuel]
78432-19-6	Dinitropyrene [see Nitropyrenes]
79217-60-0	Cyclosporine
82413-20-5	Droloxifene
82558-50-7	Isoxaben
83463-62-1	Bromochloroacetonitrile
85502-23-4	3-(N-Nitrosomethylamino)propionaldehyde
85878-62-2	Pyrido[3,4-c]psoralen
85878-63-3	7-Methylpyrido[3,4-c]-psoralen
86290-81-5	Gasoline
87625-62-5	Ptaquiloside
89778-26-7	Toremifene
90370-29-9	4,4′,6-Trimethylangelicin plus ultraviolet A radiation
90456-67-0	N-Methylolacrylamide
93763-70-3	Perlite
94624-12-1	Pentanol-1/3-Methyl butanol-1 mixture [see Pentanol, all isomers]
95481-62-2	Dicarboxylic acid (C_4–C_6) dimethyl ester, mixture
101043-37-2	Microcystin-LR
105650-23-5	2-Amino-1-methyl-6-phenylimidazo[4,5-b]pyridine [PhIP]
105735-71-5	3,7-Dinitrofluoranthene
111189-32-3	Naphtho[1,2-b]fluoranthene
112926-00-8	Silica, amorphous, precipitated and gel
116355-83-0	Fumonisin B_1
118399-22-7	Nodularins
132207-32-0	Chrysotile [see Asbestos, all forms]
136677-10-6	Polychlorinated dibenzofurans
163702-07-6	1,1,1,2,2,3,3,4,4-Nonafluoro-4-methoxybutane [see HFE-7100]
163702-08-7	2-(Difluoromethoxymethyl)-1,1,1,2,3,3,3-heptafluoropropane [see HFE-7100]
293733-21-8	6-Amino-2-ethoxynaphthalene

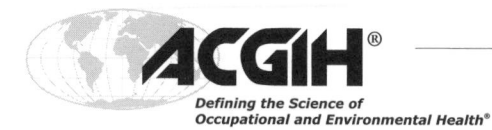

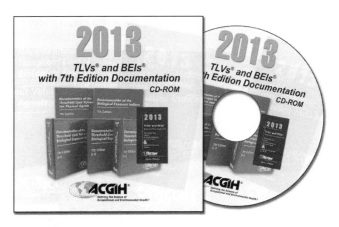
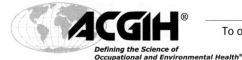

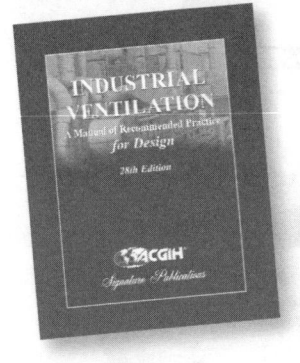
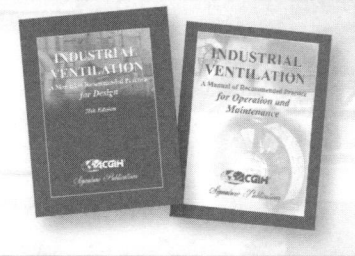
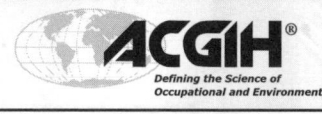

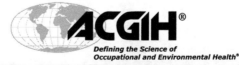

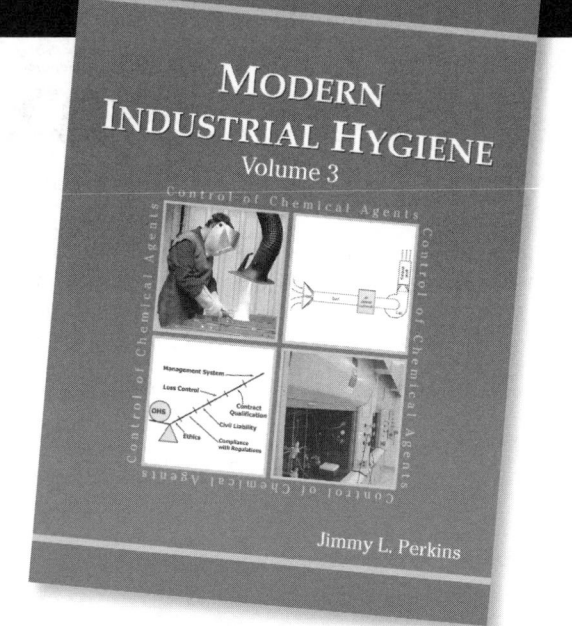
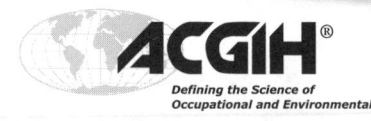

NOTES

NOTES

NOTES

NOTES

NOTES

ISBN: 978-1-607260-60-8

ISBN: 978-1-607260-60-8   © 2013

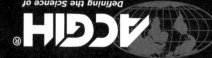

ACGIH®
Defining the Science of
Occupational and Environmental Health®

1330 Kemper Meadow Drive
Cincinnati, Ohio 45240-4148
Phone: (513)742-2020
Fax: (513)742-3355
www.acgih.org